THE ULTIMATE PALEO MEDITERRANEAN DIET

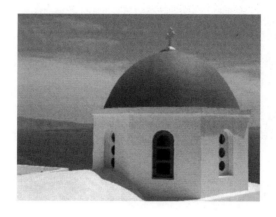

By
Mercedes del Rey

LEGAL NOTICE

The Publisher has striven to be as accurate and complete as possible in the compilation of this book.

While all attempts have been made to verify information provided in this publication, the Publisher assumes no responsibility for errors, omissions, or contrary interpretation of the subject matter herein. Any perceived slights of specific persons, peoples, or organizations are unintentional.

Additional Terms and Conditions

This book and all the information here are provided to you for information and educational purposes only. The author, creator and publisher of this guide are not medical doctors. The information contained on this site should not be construed as medical advice.

Before beginning any exercise, diet, weight loss program or treatment it is vital you contact your healthcare provider.

No warranty may be created or extended by sales representatives or written sales materials. The advice and strategies enclosed may not be suitable for your situation. You should always consult with a medical health professional when dealing with any medical condition or program involving your health and well-being. Information about health and diet cannot be generalized to the population at large. Keep in mind you should consult with a qualified physician when embarking on any program. Neither the Publisher nor Author shall be liable for any loss of profit or any other commercial damages resulting from use of this guide.

All links are for information purposes only and are not warranted for content, accuracy or any other implied or explicit purpose. No part of this publication may be reproduced, stored in a retrieval system, or transmitted in any form or by any means, electronic, mechanical, photocopying, recording, scanning, or otherwise, except as permitted under Sections 107 or 108 of the 1976 United States Copyright Act, without the prior written permission of the Publisher and Author.

Dear Reader

Thank you and congratulations on getting this book today, which contains a selection my favourite recipes. I hope that you will enjoy all of them.

My hope is that you enjoy the best possible health every single day.

Please do leave a book review if you can as this will help me in writing more of the books that you want to read and please see my other books at my Amazon Page http://amzn.to/2DGhX06

Merche

The Ultimate Paleo Mediterranean Diet By Mercedes del Rey

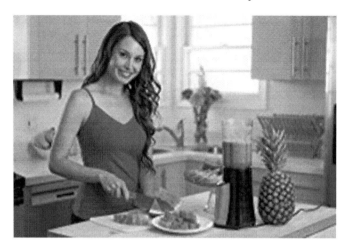

FOREWORD

Welcome to my wonderful world of completely safe and natural healing. My name is Mercedes del Rey but my friends call me Merche and I am truly fortunate to live in one of the most beautiful places in the world. My home is in sunny Andalusia in the south of Spain, the place where I was born and where I grew up before travelling to the US to complete my higher education. My life has been blessed in so many ways but I've had plenty of problems along the way.

Despite growing up in such a wonderful place, my health has not always been very strong. I suffered from a series of acute allergies throughout childhood, sometimes reacting to certain foods and then to the chemicals in ordinary household articles like hand soap and shampoo. Eventually the conditions became severe and I began my long exposure to the medical profession and a cocktail of drugs that were supposed to calm my allergies but, in the end, made my life miserable because of all the side effects. The doctors rarely mention the negative consequences of the drugs they prescribe but I felt that my condition was becoming worse rather than getting better.

There were times when I suffered from bouts of depression and a complete lack of confidence, always conscious of the rashes and marks on my skin, the unexplained outbreaks of eczema and the fear of being disfigured by the horrible discoloured patches that appeared on my face and body. In some ways, growing up was a nightmare. I turned to food as a source of comfort and then I started to gain weight, which made me feel even worse. I was highly strung, super sensitive, borderline depressed and often miserable. The drugs were no help whatsoever. And then, as if out of the blue, I met someone who turned my life around completely.

 A friend was very concerned about me. She knew I wasn't sleeping well, that my allergies were a constant source of discomfort and embarrassment, that I was depressed and that I'd hit a low spot in my life where i no longer knew where to turn for help. She recommended someone to me, a very special person, a lady who understood exactly what was wrong with me and who showed me how to change my life forever using the most natural remedies imaginable. Her name is Beran Parry and her knowledge of herbalism opened my life to an extraordinary world of natural healing. Beran has a very wide knowledge and experience of health, nutrition and all the factors that can contribute to complete wellbeing. The results of her advice and guidance were simply astonishing. My allergies have disappeared. My mood swings have vanished. I sleep wonderfully, and my confidence has soared. I was so impressed with her knowledge that I became her pupil and studied with her years. She has inspired me to travel the world on my quest to research and investigate herbal medicine and all that it entails.

I visited China, India, Germany, USA and Canada and met with so many wonderful Naturopathic Doctors and Herbalists along my learning path.

I now practice as an Holistic Nutritionist and I advise my own clients on the use and application of herbal remedies. It was Beran, of course, who encouraged me to write this book and she assisted me with my research. My dearest hope is that it proves to be as useful and helpful to you as her teaching has been to me.

This is not a medical advice book so please always check any remedy with your medical and naturopathic doctor at all times!

May the force of Nature be with you!

TABLE CONTENTS

The Ultimate Paleo Mediterranean Diet By Mercedes del Rey

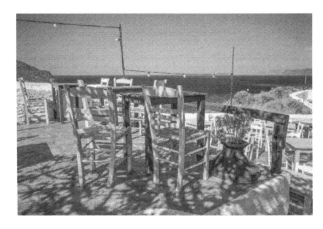

Welcome to a wonderfully wholesome approach to feeling incredibly well! Let's start by emphasizing that your new, health-enhancing way of eating certainly does not have to be either bland or boring. We're going to be working with some of the most delicious recipes you've ever tasted, sharing the great news that healthy eating can be one of the tastiest ways to burn off excess weight, relieve a long list of stubborn health conditions and boost both your energy and your quality of life. And you get to enjoy every mouthful! It really can be a pleasure to eat well and use these exciting recipes to take the very best care of your body.

Mediterranean Paleo Cooking combines the joy of Mediterranean cooking with the health-enhancing benefits of the famous Paleo Diet system. We've listened carefully to our bodies and banished gluten, grains, harmful oils, dairy products and those deadly, refined sweeteners. The Mediterranean Diet features an amazing variety of dishes from the sun-kissed shores of southern Europe, North Africa and the Levant and combines them with the health-boosting benefits of the incredibly effective Paleo diet. We've combed these regions to pick out over 150 stunning recipes, adding two 30-day meal plans (one that has been designed for total physical health and one that has been crafted for individuals who are following auto-immune diets), shopping lists, cooking tips and plenty of helpful material. Mediterranean Paleo Cooking has been designed to bring a sense of fun and enjoyment into the kitchen, teaching you how to become more proficient around the stove and transforming smart, healthy eating into a completely delicious eating experience that the whole family can enjoy every single day.

WHAT IS THE MEDITERRANEAN DIET?

The Mediterranean diet is based on the traditional food that is prepared and consumed every day in the Mediterranean area of southern Europe. The diet focuses on plentiful servings of vegetables, whole grains and beans. Seafood is usually included as a staple twice a week and limited amounts of dairy and eggs also feature in the diet. One of the advantages of the Mediterranean Diet is that red meat and sugar are avoided, and alcohol consumption is surprisingly limited, although red wine is consumed in moderation. Spices often take the place of salt, and olive oil is widely used as a substitute for butter. As you might expect in a healthy diet, Mediterranean cuisine is high in fiber, antioxidants and lots of healthy fats such as the essential omega-3 fatty acids. Mono-unsaturated fats like virgin olive oils are widely used. the Mediterranean diet favours dairy products such as cheese and yogurt but it limits eggs to around four per week. For dessert, they prefer the simple pleasures of fresh fruit. Beans and legumes are favored, using lentils and chickpeas dishes like hummus. The Mediterranean diet gained in popularity during the 1990s when it was promoted by Dr. Ancel Key, an American living in Italy at the time.

One of the surprising benefits of the Mediterranean diet that is fully supported by extensive research is that it can improve brain and memory function by around twenty percent. It reduces mental decay and promotes better cognitive awareness. The Mediterranean diet has been widely celebrated as an effective method to prevent heart disease and encourage weight loss, but it has also been shown to increase longevity and act as a preventative agent against depression.

The Paleo Mediterranean Approach to Eating. Not a diet but a way of life

Dieting and weight loss have become a multi-billion Dollar industry that tempts desperate people to part with their cash in return for the promise of an elusive and often disappointing dream. The adverts and promises are everywhere. But how many of these diets actually work? The evidence suggests that the majority of dieters experience the initial loss of a few pounds but almost inevitably pile the weight back on as soon as they take a break from the diet regime. That's why we don't need another fad diet. What we need is a smart nutritional approach that succeeds in burning off the unwanted weight and maintains a healthier, slimmer and fitter silhouette by respecting exactly what the body needs in terms of perfectly balanced food. That's where the Paleo Mediterranean approach provides the ideal combination of dietary principles to maintain a stronger, fitter, slimmer and healthier body.

We're living in a world where obesity rates are soaring and the increase in serious disease rates has become truly alarming. And one of the common denominators for these disturbing phenomena is our diet. Learning to adopt a healthy diet is the most fundamental step towards transforming your physical, mental and emotional wellness. Unhealthy dietary habits are widely responsible for the development of some of the most serious health conditions in the US today, diseases that include heart disease, cancer and diabetes. The Paleo and Mediterranean approaches to food choice equally encourage healthy eating as a way of life. There are many well-researched benefits to this fabulous approach to eating healthily.

Mediterranean Diet Basics

The Mediterranean diet has a long and well-researched heritage. Travelers, for example, have been noting the health and longevity of the peoples living around the Mediterranean for hundreds of years. And it's always worth reminding ourselves that the food from this region tastes divine. Greek and Italian cuisine has rightly been associated with fantastic flavors, culinary creativity and the kind of robust vitality that flows from a naturally healthy diet. The basics are very easy to learn:

The Ultimate Paleo Mediterranean Diet By Mercedes del Rey

1.   The old ideas of our grandparents often contained the benefit of very sound advice. So, you should aim to eat three normal meals per day with a gap of around five hours between each sitting. This is very helpful for maintaining normal blood sugar levels. Never eat carbohydrates on their own. It's important to add a measure of protein to your meals and snacks. It is particularly helpful to avoid a carbohydrate-only breakfast and to keep overall carbs to around 15-20 gm per meal. Put the odds on your side. Develop the enjoyable habit of shopping for fresh whole food. Enjoy your food by chewing thoroughly and pausing between bites to savor the flavor. Banish the habit of eating after the evening meal.

2.   Cut out the unhealthy stimulants such as caffeine, sugar, alcohol and tobacco. Stimulants encourage the stress-response system to release epinephrine and cortisol which raises blood sugar to release energy.

3.   Stop eating all forms of junk food. These empty calories only harm the body's health and cannot contribute to the development of a healthy body.

4.   Remove all trans-fats from your food choices. Cell membranes, nerve tissue and steroid hormones require healthy fats in order to function normally. Unhealthy fats, that occur in so many processed foods, interfere with these vital physical functions.

5.   Make a decision to eat unprocessed, whole, fresh food. Minimize fruit juices since they contain far too much sugar, even though many people mistakenly believe that fruit sugar is somehow better than processed sugar.

6.   Use plenty of sea salt in your cooking and on your food. The glands that are responsible for handling stress-handling need salt for normal functioning. Research has shown that salt does NOT contribute to high blood pressure or heart disease. Only people with organ damage, such as kidney disease, need to follow a low-salt diet. In fact, low-salt diets can increase adrenal fatigue.

7.   Drink plenty of water (pure, filtered or spring water, but not tap water).

Other benefits of the Mediterranean diet

One of the other well-publicized benefits of the Mediterranean diet is a reduction in the occurrence of strokes. Extensive research has revealed that people who observe this healthy lifestyle choice in their nutrition enjoy a better health-related quality of life (HRQL). This improvement in health has been attributed to the organic increase in dietary fiber and the prevalence of antioxidants. Additional research has demonstrated that the Mediterranean diet is clearly beneficial for overall heart health. Scientists and doctors have shown that this lifestyle choice can slow down the effects of aging, reduce the risk of stroke and the cut the risk of contracting endometrial cancer. Some researchers have concluded that the diet can prevent diabetes, but this is inconclusive, because the consumption of complex carbohydrates is not considered beneficial for those with insulin resistance or metabolic syndrome.

The Ultimate Paleo Mediterranean Diet By Mercedes del Rey

Osteoporosis is a condition that most people happily ignore until it becomes a health problem and this is something that usually occurs later in life. Whilst both men and women can experience this disturbing weakening of the bones, it is a particular issue for women, especially after the onset of menopause. The reduction in estrogen levels associated with menopause can often lead to calcium loss from the bones. This is the common origin of brittle bones in older people. Brittle bones can obviously lead to an increase in risk of serious fractures, including fractures of the hip which can lead to a permanent loss of mobility and the essential sense of independence that helps older people thrive in later life.

Happily, women who consume higher quantities of olive oil have a reduced risk of developing weakened or brittle bones. And there is intriguing evidence that supports a link between bone strength and olive oil consumption.

Olive oil and the Mediterranean diet

Is there a link between olive oil consumption and bone strength? We know that women in Mediterranean countries typically consume a diet that is rich in fresh fruits and vegetables and, perhaps more importantly, a diet that is also rich in olive oil. That equates to at least 2-4 tablespoons daily. The kind of olive oil that is widely preferred also happens to be the richest in nutrients and that means extra virgin and first-pressed. This is the kind of first class olive oil that is good for general health and for maintaining great bone strength.

These vitally important health benefits are the result the presence of potent antioxidant compounds. These compounds reduce inflammation throughout the body, lower cholesterol levels, prevent oxidative stress to the cells and reduce the chances of heart attacks and strokes. It is also believed that regular consumption of olive oil can help lower the risk of certain cancers, particularly of the colon.

Mediterranean diet slows cellular aging, study shows

If you're interested in your own longevity, we may have the answer to your quest in the nature of the food you eat. That's right. According to a recent study published in the British Medical Journal, people simply need to subscribe to the Mediterranean diet and they will significantly increase their chances to live longer, healthier lives.

Researchers in the US have demonstrated that the Mediterranean diet, which primarily focuses on fresh fish, fruits, olive oil and vegetables, helps to promote longer telomere length. Why is this important? A longer telomere length plays an essential role in protecting the chromosomes in our DNA from losing genetic information, data that is typically lost as a result of the aging process. Cell decay and death and shorter telomere are closely connected. They often provide an indicator of an increased likelihood of developing heart disease, high blood pressure and strokes.

Largest population-based study reinforces benefits of Mediterranean diet

The findings were part of an ongoing study going back to the 1970s that ultimately assessed over 5,000 healthy, middle-aged women. Blood tests and questionnaires based on their dietary lifestyle ultimately showed that those enjoying a Mediterranean diet tended to have longer telomeres. This showed that the diet was an important factor in slowing cellular aging.

"To our knowledge, this is the largest population-based study specifically addressing the association between Mediterranean diet adherence and telomere length in healthy, middle-aged women," the researchers noted. "Our results further support the benefits of adherence to the Mediterranean diet for promoting health and longevity." The authors wrote that " ... greater adherence to the Mediterranean diet was significantly associated with longer leukocyte telomere length, a marker of biological aging. Our results further support the health benefits of adherence to the Mediterranean diet."

The Mediterranean approach to eating

Unlike many fad diets and short-term approaches to supposedly balanced and healthy eating, the Mediterranean Diet allows for a very wide variety of unprocessed whole foods, as long as moderation is practised as the cardinal rule. There's very little consumption of sugary pastries or other sweets, but whole grains can be consumed daily. However, as you might expect, there are important differences between the southern European approach to baking and the typical American way of preparing grains. Traditional baking includes slower fermentation without rushing and baking without bromides or other toxic additives and preservatives. Pasta and couscous are also more natural and they form a normal part of the daily diet. Bleaching flours with chemicals is usually considered unnatural.

Fish, especially shell fish, dominate the animal protein menu and they are rarely exposed to batter or fried. Lean meats are permitted but always in moderation.

Similarities and Differences

The Paleo and Mediterranean diets both highlight fish as optimal sources of protein and omega-3 fatty acids. Limiting the amount of saturated fat in your diet is one crucial component for promoting heart health and both diets encourage several daily servings of fresh fruits and vegetables for getting the vitamins, nutrients and antioxidants required to maintain health and prevent disease. The diets also favor nuts, seeds olive oil for flavoring rather than using fatty dressings. The diets differ in the consumption of dairy foods and of grain products like breads, pastas and cereals. MayoClinic.com notes that the Mediterranean diet encourages eating low-fat dairy to maintain calcium, vitamin D and protein needs. Whole grains are equally important to provide fiber for healthy digestion and keeping cholesterol levels lower.

Benefits of Paleo-Mediterranean Dieting

According to a 2009 pilot study in "Cardiovascular Diabetology," diabetic participants placed on a Paleo diet showed improved blood sugar control and reduced risk for cardiovascular disorders compared to eating a diabetic diet alone. Similarly, the "British Medical Journal" published a 2008 study of non-diabetic participants on a Mediterranean style diet that had a 35 percent reduction in risk for developing diabetes due to changing eating patterns. The crux of choosing a Paleo or Mediterranean diet lies in limiting foods with saturated fats and refined sugars while also increasing consumption of raw produce that promotes arterial health and normal digestion. Both diets offer benefits for cardiovascular health, prevention or management of glucose-related disorders and a means for consuming foods that may protect against forms of cancer. Choose the right nutritional plan based on your current health status and recommendations from your physician.

Mediterranean Paleo Cooking helps readers become better cooks and more informed eaters. But more importantly, it turns healthy eating into delicious eating with enticing Mediterranean meals that every foodie will enjoy.

RECIPES

BREAKFAST

1. Breakfast Sweet Potato Hash

Ingredients

1 large onion, sliced

3 tbsp olive oil, divided

1/2 tbsp ghee

2 Italian sausages, diced

2 sweet potatoes

3 tbsp fresh rosemary

Salt and freshly ground black pepper, to taste

3 eggs

Instructions

Preheat the oven to 425 degrees F. Line a baking sheet with parchment paper. Heat one tablespoon of olive oil and the ghee in a skillet over medium heat. Add the onions and sprinkle with salt. Cook on low heat for 30-40 minutes, until dark brown and caramelized.

Meanwhile, peel the sweet potatoes and chop into bite-size pieces. Place into a large bowl with the remaining two tablespoons of olive oil and rosemary.

In a separate skillet, cook the sausages until browned. Add the cooked onions and sausages to the bowl with the sweet potatoes and toss. Season with salt and pepper.

Spread out the sweet potato mixture evenly onto the prepared baking sheet. Roast for 30-35 minutes until the potatoes are soft and browned. Either refrigerate overnight at this point or proceed to the next step.

Place the sweet potato hash into a cast iron skillet and make three small wells to crack the eggs into. Crack eggs into the skillet and season lightly with salt and pepper. Bake for 15-18 minutes at 425 degrees F until the eggs are set.

Notes

Servings: 4

Difficulty: Medium

⁂

2.   Mile High Power Breakfast Burger

Ingredients

To make the patties, you will need:

450g grass fed ground beef

1/3 cup crispy lardons (or 2-3 crispy bacon strips and their drippings)

1 tbsp Dijon mustard

3 cloves garlic, chopped

1 pastured egg

¼ tsp Himalayan or unrefined sea salt

¼ tsp freshly cracked black pepper

¼ tsp anise seeds

1/8 tsp ground clove

1 large jalapeño pepper, seeded and very finely chopped

¼ cup fresh parsley, finely chopped

2 tbsp fresh mint, finely chopped

1 tbsp fresh rosemary, finely chopped

½ cup sauerkraut, squeezed fairly dry and roughly chopped

To garnish each burger, you will need:

1 fresh kale leaf, torn into several pieces

2 slices tomato

3 slices avocado

¼ cup sauerkraut

1 pastured egg, pan fried

1 bacon strip, cooked and cut in 2 pieces

Instructions

Start by cooking the required number of slices of bacon (depending on how many burgers you are making and whether or not you are using cooked bacon in your meat patties) and set aside.

In a small food processor, add the lardons (or cooked bacon and drippings) Dijon mustard, garlic, egg, salt, pepper, ground clove and anise seeds and process into a paste.

Add that to a medium mixing bowl along with the ground beef, jalapeño pepper, parsley, mint, rosemary and sauerkraut and knead well with your hands until uniformly blended. Form the meat mixture into 3 or 4 beef patties.

Preheat your outdoor grill to high.

Once your grill is nice and hot, lower the heat to medium and place the patties on the grill; cook for about 3-4 minutes per side or until the patties are done to your liking.

Alternatively, you could also cook the beef patties in a large skillet set over medium-high heat, again, about 3-4 minutes per side.

While the meat is cooking, pan fry as many eggs as you will require to garnish your burgers.

To assemble the burgers, start by laying a few pieces of kale at the bottom of a plate. Place the beef patty right over that, followed by the sauerkraut and a few slices of tomatoes and avocado.

At this point, you might want to insert a toothpick right in the center of the pile to make sure your mile high burger doesn't collapse on you!

Once everything is good and secure, add the pan fried egg right on top of all that and, finally, place two pieces of cooked bacon right over your egg. BEAUTY!

Take a nice long look (if you can!) at your beautiful creation and dig in.

⁇

3.   Paleo Garlic Breadsticks (Just Don't Eat Them All Yourself)

Ingredients
1 1/3 cups almond flour
1/2 tsp salt
2 tbsp coconut oil, melted
3 tbsp coconut flour
1 clove garlic, minced
3 eggs, divided
1 tsp dried basil
1/2 tsp onion powder
1/2 tsp oregano
1/2 tsp baking powder
Ghee, for brushing

Instructions
Whisk two eggs together in a small bowl and set aside. In a separate bowl, add the almond flour, baking powder, salt, and coconut oil and stir. Add the beaten eggs and stir to combine.
Add the coconut flour into the bowl, one tablespoon at a time. After each tablespoon let the dough rest for a minute as the flour absorbs. Add the next tablespoon and repeat until you have dough that can be easily kneaded.
Preheat the oven to 350 degrees F. Line a baking sheet with parchment paper. Roll out the dough onto a separate piece of parchment paper. Working in small handfuls, roll the dough into a long rope. Twist the dough into your shape of choice and place on the baking sheet. Bake for 10 minutes.
Whisk the remaining egg and add a dash of water. Remove the breadsticks from the oven and brush with the egg wash, and then the minced garlic, basil, onion powder and oregano. Return to the oven and bake for 4-5 minutes more, until golden. Brush with melted ghee before serving.

Notes
Servings: 4-8 breadsticks, depending on size
Difficulty: Medium
⏲

4. Homemade Strawberry Fruit Leather

Ingredients
4 cups strawberries, hulled and chopped
2 tbsp honey

Instructions
Preheat the oven to 170 degrees F or the lowest oven temperature setting. Line a baking sheet with a Silpat mat. Place strawberries in a medium saucepan and cook on low heat until soft. Add in the honey and stir to combine.

Use an immersion blender to puree the strawberries in the saucepan, or transfer to a blender and puree until smooth. Pour the mixture onto the Silpat-lined baking sheet and spread evenly with a spatula. Bake for 6-7 hours, until it peels away from the parchment.

Once cooled, peel the fruit leather off the mat and use a scissors to cut the fruit leather into strips. Roll up to serve, and store in an airtight container.

Notes
Servings: approximately 12 strips
Difficulty: Medium
?

5.   Spicy Southwestern Breakfast Bowl

Ingredients
2 large sweet potatoes, peeled and diced
Extra virgin olive oil, for drizzling
Salt and pepper, to taste
1 tsp chili powder
2 strips bacon
1/2 medium yellow onion, diced
1/2 green bell pepper, diced
1/2 red bell pepper, diced
1 small jalapeno, seeded and diced
2-3 cups fresh spinach
2 eggs
1 tsp ghee
1 avocado, pitted and diced, optional

Instructions
Preheat the oven to 375 degrees F. Place the diced sweet potatoes on a rimmed baking sheet and drizzle with olive oil. Sprinkle with salt, pepper, and chili powder. Bake for 15-20 minutes, turning once. Meanwhile, cook the bacon in a skillet over medium heat. Remove to a paper towel-lined plate and crumble. Add the onion, bell peppers, and jalapeno to the skillet and sauté for 5-6 minutes until soft. Lastly add in the spinach and cook until wilted.
In a separate skillet, melt the ghee. Cook the eggs to desired doneness, seasoning with salt and pepper.
To assemble, divide the sweet potatoes between two bowls. Top with the veggie mixture, followed by the egg, crumbled bacon, and avocado if using.

Notes
Servings: 2
Difficulty: Easy
⬚

6.   Down-Home Brussels Sprout Hash

Ingredients
3 slices bacon
1/2 large butternut squash, peeled, seeded and cubed
1/2 small red onion, finely diced
1 clove garlic, minced
12 oz. Brussels sprouts, stemmed and sliced
1 tbsp extra virgin olive oil
Salt and freshly ground pepper, to taste
2-3 eggs, optional

Instructions
Place the bacon in a pan and cook until crisp. Set aside on a paper towel-lined plate and crumble into pieces. Leave one tablespoon of bacon grease in the pan and dispose of the rest.
Add the butternut squash, onion, and garlic to the pan and cook for 5-7 minutes, stirring occasionally, until soft. Stir in the Brussels sprouts, along with a tablespoon of olive oil. Season generously with salt and pepper to taste. Sauté for 8-10 minutes until the Brussels sprouts are bright green and fork-tender.
Add the crumbled bacon back into the pan and stir. Make two or three small wells in the hash and crack an egg into each. Cover and cook until the eggs are set. Serve immediately.

Notes
Servings: 2-3
Difficulty: Easy
⁇

7.   Paleo Stuffed Breakfast Peppers

Ingredients
2 bell peppers – your choice of colour
4 eggs
1 cup white mushrooms
1 cup broccoli
¼ tsp cayenne pepper
Salt and pepper, to taste

Instructions
Preheat oven to 375 degrees Fahrenheit.
Dice up your vegetables of choice.
In a medium sized bowl, mix eggs, salt, pepper, cayenne pepper, and vegetables.
Cut peppers into equal halves. A tip: Try to buy peppers that are symmetrical and have somewhat flat sides – this makes it easier for them to balance while baking.
Core the peppers so that they're clean enough to add the filling.
Pour a quarter of the egg / vegetable mix into each pepper halve, adding more vegetables to the top to fill in any empty space.
Place on baking sheet and cook approximately 35 minutes or until eggs are cooked to your liking.
Serve and enjoy! I personally like mine with a dash of hot sauce on top.

Notes
This recipe makes 2 servings.
Nutrition Facts Per Serving
Calories: 186
Total Fat: 9.4g
Saturated Fat: 2.8g
Carbs: 12.1g
Fiber: 4.0g
Protein: 14.6g

8. Breakfast Quiche with Broccoli and Ham

Ingredients

3 tbsp of water

8 eggs

1 tsp of sea salt

1 tsp of black pepper

2 cups of broccoli chopped small

2 cups of red onions

2 cups of ham

1 tsp of coconut oil

Instructions

Bake pie dish for 5 minutes on 350 degrees fahrenheit.

Lightly steam broccoli for a couple of minutes, should turn a pretty bright green. Set aside.

Saute chopped red onions and chopped ham in coconut oil. If ham is fatty skip coconut oil, the fat will render and be enough.

Add veggies to lightly baked pie crust.

Then whisk eggs and water and add over veggies. Water helps make eggs fluffy, so does baking soda. Other recipes I googled use almond and coconut milk. Your pick.

Bake for 25-30 minutes or until desired firmness.

Notes

Tip: I always undercook food, you can always put it in the oven for longer.

Nutrition Information

Serving size: 4-6

☐

9.   Healthy Low Carb Crustless Quiche Recipe

Ingredients
6 organic, free range eggs
6 stalks kale
6 stalks swiss chard
15 campari tomatoes, 10 cut into quarters and 5 with stem attached
2 medium shallots sliced thin, or half a sweet onion, diced
1 Tbs whole grain mustard
1 tsp garlic powder
1/4 tsp red pepper flakes – use more or less to taste
4 oz shredded parmesan cheese
1 Tbs organic butter
salt and pepper

Instructions
Preheat your oven to 350 degrees F (175 degrees C).
In a nonstick skillet over med-high heat, melt your butter. Add shallots and a little salt and pepper and cook until translucent, about 2 mins.
Grab your kale and swiss chard by the stem and strip the leaves from the stem with your hands. (I like to save the stems and use them later in my veggie juices)! Again, using your hands, tear the leaves into small pieces and add to your skillet. Next add your tomatoes, mustard, red pepper flakes, and more salt & pepper. Using a wooden spoon, stir all ingredients together, taste and adjust spices as needed, and remove from heat.
Whisk eggs and parmesan in a large bowl until well combined. Pour the egg mixture into your skillet and stir to combine with the vegetables. Then top with your tomatoes on the vine. You could also transfer all of your ingredients into a baking or pie dish, but I like to keep it simple so I bake the dish in the same skillet; just remember to use an oven mitt to remove from the oven!
Bake until golden brown and eggs are completely set, about 30- 35 mins. Allow quiche to cool for 10 minutes before serving.
⁇

10.   Sun-Dried Tomato Quiche

Ingredients
5 eggs
1 zucchini
1 onion
¼ tsp salt
¼ tsp pepper
2 tsp coconut oil
2 tomatoes, small
4 oz sundried tomatoes
¼ lb pancetta, sliced

Instructions
Preheat oven to 350° F.
Grease an 8-inch cast-iron skillet with 1 tsp coconut oil and set aside.
Melt 1 tsp coconut oil in a medium skillet over medium heat. Whirl the onion and zucchini in a food processor until finely shredded, then cook in the skillet until soft and translucent, about 10 minutes.
While the zucchini and onions soften, drain the oil from your sun-dried tomatoes if you're using oil-packed. Roughly chop and add to a medium mixing bowl.
Pull the pancetta slices apart with your fingers into shreds, then add to the tomatoes.
When the onions and zucchini are soft, add to the pancetta and tomatoes. Mix thoroughly and allow to cool to room temperature. Whisk in eggs, salt and pepper and pour into the cast-iron skillet.
Cook in the preheated oven for 1 hour and 15 minutes or until firm.
Serve warm.
⯑

11. Paleo Breakfast Burritos (Low-Carb)

Ingredients
For the tortillas
2 eggs
2 egg whites
1/2 cup water
4 tsp ground flaxseed
Pinch of salt

For the filling
1 avocado, diced
1/4 cup red bell pepper, finely diced
1/4 cup onion, finely diced
1/4 cup baked tilapia or other protein
Handful of spinach leaves
1 tsp coconut oil

Instructions
In a small bowl, whisk together the ingredients for the tortilla. Preheat the oven broiler.
Heat a 10-inch non-stick skillet over medium heat and coat well with coconut oil spray. Pour half of the tortilla mixture into the pan and swirl to evenly distribute. Using a metal spatula, loosen the edges of the tortilla from the pan. Cook a couple of minutes until golden brown on the bottom, and then carefully slide the spatula under the tortilla to loosen it from the bottom of the pan. Do not flip yet.
Place the pan under the broiler for 3-4 minutes until the tortilla gets a little bubbly. Remove the tortilla from the pan, setting on a piece of aluminium foil. Repeat with other half of tortilla mixture.
After the tortillas are done broiling, preheat the oven to 400 degrees F. In a separate small pan, heat the coconut oil over medium heat. Add the onions and peppers and sauté for 5-8 minutes, until soft. Add the spinach into the pan and wilt.
Place all of the fillings down the center of the tortillas and wrap tightly. Place into the oven for 5-8 minutes to set the shape of the tortilla. Enjoy!
Notes
Servings: 2
Difficulty: Medium
☐

12.   Homemade Strawberry Fruit Leather

Ingredients
4 cups strawberries, hulled and chopped
2 tbsp honey

Instructions
Preheat the oven to 170 degrees F or the lowest oven temperature setting. Line a baking sheet with a Silpat mat. Place strawberries in a medium saucepan and cook on low heat until soft. Add in the honey and stir to combine.

Use an immersion blender to puree the strawberries in the saucepan, or transfer to a blender and puree until smooth. Pour the mixture onto the Silpat-lined baking sheet and spread evenly with a spatula. Bake for 6-7 hours, until it peels away from the parchment.

Once cooled, peel the fruit leather off the mat and use a scissors to cut the fruit leather into strips. Roll up to serve, and store in an airtight container.

Notes
Servings: approximately 12 strips
Difficulty: Medium
?

LUNCH

13.   Tuna Avocado Lettuce Wraps (Makes the Perfect Lunch)

Ingredients
1 can tuna
½ very ripe avocado
2 tbsp paleo mayo
¼ cup green olives
2 tbsp diced green chillies
1 scallion
2 large leaves of green leaf lettuce (or your favourite green!)
This recipe serves two, but is so good you just may eat the whole thing yourself.

Instructions
Cut olives in half and dice scallion.
Mash the avocado until it's a creamy consistency, and then mix with paleo mayonnaise.
Add in the tuna, olives, scallion, and diced green chillies to the avocado-mayonnaise mixture.
Place one scoop of tuna salad into a large leaf of lettuce, wrap, and enjoy!
⁇

14. Low Carb Chipotle Chicken Lettuce Wraps

Ingredients
2 tbsp extra virgin olive oil
1 lb. boneless skinless chicken breast
3 chipotle peppers
4 tbsp adobo sauce
1/3 cup cilantro, chopped
Juice of 1 lime
1/2 red bell pepper, diced
2 scallions, thinly sliced
1 head lettuce, rinsed
Salt and freshly ground pepper

Instructions
Heat the olive oil in a large pan over medium heat. Sprinkle the chicken with salt and pepper on both sides and place in the pan. Cook for 5-6 minutes per side until the chicken is cooked through. Set aside and rest for 5 minutes, then shred.

In a food processor or blender, combine the chipotle peppers, adobo, cilantro, and lime juice. Blend until smooth.

Add the bell pepper, adobo mixture, and chicken to the sauté pan on low heat. Stir well to combine and cook for 3-4 minutes. Add the scallions to the pan. Spoon the mixture into lettuce wraps and serve.

Notes
Servings: 6-8 wraps
Difficulty: Medium
⁇

15.   Fennel and Brussels Sprouts Sirloin Rolls

Ingredients
For the Filling:
2 slices bacon, chopped into 4 or 5 large pieces
½ fennel bulb, roughly chopped
1/2 cup Brussels sprouts, bottoms trimmed off and halved
2 garlic cloves
1 tsp each of dried rosemary, sage and oregano

Additional Ingredient:
2½ lb sirloin steaks
Salt and pepper, to taste
2 cups Brussels sprouts (about ¾ lb), bottoms trimmed off and quartered
½ fennel bulb, cut into thick slices
1 tsp olive oil
2 or 3 fennel fronds

Instructions
Preheat oven to 375F.
Add all filling ingredients to a food processor. Process until it forms a thick paste.
Pound out steaks using a mallet until they are about ½ inch thick.
Spread half of the filling on each steak. Roll steaks up, using a few toothpicks to secure.
Place sirloin rolls in a large roasting pan and sprinkle with salt and pepper.
Toss Brussels sprouts and fennel slices in a large bowl with olive oil, salt and pepper.
Spread Brussels sprouts and fennel slices around sirloin rolls in the roasting pan.
Roast for 35-40 minutes, until steak is cooked to desired level and vegetables begin to brown. If steak is done and veggies need to cook a bit longer, remove the steak from the pan and let it rest while you cook the veggies for an additional five minutes or so.
Let steak rest for 5 minutes before slicing. Garnish with fennel fronds.
▢

16.   Tasty Testy Lettuce Wraparounds

Ingredients

8 oz skinless, boneless chicken or turkey ground

1/4 cup water chestnuts, chopped fine

1/4 cup dried shiitake mushrooms

1 tbsp soy sauce (I used reduced sodium)

1 1/2 tsp sesame oil

1 tsp rice wine or dry sherry

1/2 tsp stevia

freshly ground white pepper, to taste

2 cloves garlic, finely chopped

6 large iceberg lettuce leaves, rinsed)

2 tbsp diced scallions

Instructions

Place mushrooms in hot water to soften a few minutes. Remove stems and chop fine.

Combine all sauces and dry ingredients in a bowl.

Combine ground chicken mushrooms and water chestnuts into a bowl. Pour over chicken; toss. Let marinate for 15 minutes.

Heat remaining sesame oil in a wok or skillet over high heat. Add garlic; cook until golden, about 10 seconds. Add chicken mixture; stir fry until browned, breaking the chicken up as it cooks, about 4-5 minutes.

To serve, spoon 1/4 cup of the mixture into each lettuce leaf. Garnish with scallions

☐

17.   Pumpkin Avocado Salad

Ingredients
2 tbsp red onion, chopped
2 tbsp lime juice
2 medium hass avocados, diced
2 cups cooked pumpkin, diced
2 tbsp chopped cilantro
Low sodium salt and pepper to taste

Instructions
In a small bowl combine onion, lime juice and low sodium salt.
In a medium bowl, combine avocados, pumpkin, and cilantro. Toss with lime juice and onions and serve immediately.
⁇

18.   Punchy Tomato Salsa

Ingredients
4 medium ripe tomatoes, chopped
1/4 cup finely chopped white onion
2 chilli peppers, mild or hot, seeded and finely chopped
2 tbsps chopped bell pepper
1 clove garlic, minced
1/4 cup finely chopped fresh cilantro leaves (no stems)
2 tbsps fresh lime juice
Low sodium salt and pepper, to taste

Instructions
In a bowl combine all ingredients. Let it marinate in the refrigerator at least an hour for best results.
⁇

19.   Sexy Salsa

Ingredients
3 medium tomatoes, cored and quartered
1 jalapeño, stem removed and roasted
3-4 small cloves garlic
2 tbsp cilantro
3-4 tbsp water
1 tsp olive oil
Low sodium salt to taste

Instructions
In a blender, add tomatoes, jalapeño, garlic, cilantro and water and pulse a few times until completely smooth.
Add oil to a deep skillet, then pour in tomatoes. Season with low sodium salt and simmer uncovered stirring occasionally, 20 to 25 minutes.
⯑

20.   Crispy Chicken Wings

Ingredients

3 lbs (about 18) chicken wings

1/4 cup white vinegar

2 tbsp oregano

4 tsp paprika

1 tbsp garlic powder

1 tbsp chili powder

Low sodium salt and fresh pepper

2 celery stalks, sliced into strips

2 carrots, peeled and sliced into strips

Instructions

In a large bowl combine chicken, vinegar, oregano, paprika, garlic powder, chili powder salt and pepper. Mix well and let marinate for 30 minutes.

Place wings on a broiler rack and broil on low, about 8 inches from the flame for about 10-12 minutes on each side

While chicken cooks, heat the remaining hot sauce until warm. Toss the hot sauce with the chicken and arrange on a platter. Serve with celery and carrot strips.

▢

21.   Sexy Prawn Salsa

Ingredients

16 oz cooked peeled prawns diced in large chunks

4 vine ripe tomatoes, diced fine

6 tbsp red onion, finely diced

2 tbsp minced cilantro

2 limes, juice of (or more to taste)

1/2 tsp low sodium salt

Instructions

Combine diced onions, tomatoes, salt and lime juice in a non-reactive bowl and let it sit about 5 minutes.

Combine the remaining ingredients in a large bowl, taste for low sodium salt and adjust as needed.

Refrigerate and let the flavours combine at least an hour before serving.

?

22. Divine Juicy Tuna Sashimi

Ingredients

8 oz sushi grade tuna, finely chopped

2 tsps pure sesame oil

1 tsp rice wine

2 tsp fresh lime juice

2 tsplow sodium gluten free soy sauce

1 ripe, firm hass avocado, diced

1 tsp black and white sesame seeds

Instructions

Combine sesame oil, lime juice, soy sauce. . Pour over tuna and mix. Add chives and gently combine tuna with diced avocado, refrigerate until ready to serve….top with sesame seeds.

⁇

23.   Steamed Brussels Mussels with Fresh Basil

Ingredients

2 dozen mussels

2 tsp olive oil

3 cloves garlic, cut in large chunks

2 tbsp fresh herbs such as basil or parsley

1/tblspn white wine

1/4 cup water

Instructions

Heat a large pot on high heat. Add oil. When hot, add garlic and cook until golden.

Add wine, water and mussels and cover tightly, reduce to medium-low heat.

Cook 5 to 10 minutes, or until the shells open. Do not overcook or the mussels will become rubbery.

Transfer with a slotted spoon to a large bowl and pour the liquid through a strainer over the clams. Top with fresh herbs and enjoy.

[?]

24.   Summer Tuna and Avocado Salad

Ingredients

2 tins albacore tuna in water ..low salt

1 pint grape tomatoes, cut in half

1 hass avocado, diced

2 hot peppers such as serrano or jalapeños, diced fine (seeds removed for mild)

1/3 cup chopped red onion

2 limes, juice of (or more to taste)

1 tsp olive oil

2 tbsps chopped cilantro

Low sodium salt and fresh pepper to taste

Instructions

In a small bowl combine red onion, lime juice, olive oil, pinch of low sodium salt and pepper. Let them marinate at least 5 minutes to mellow the flavour of the onion.

In a large bowl combine tuna, avocado, tomatoes, hot pepper Combine all the ingredients together, add cilantro and gently toss. Adjust lime juice, low sodium salt and pepper to taste.

25. Mediterranean Supercharger Omelet with Fennel and Dill

Ingredients

2 tablespoons olive oil, divided

2 cups thinly sliced fresh fennel bulb, fronds chopped and reserved

8 cherry tomatoes

5 large eggs, beaten to blend with 1/4 teaspoon salt and 1/4 teaspoon ground black pepper

1 1/2 tablespoons chopped fresh dill

Instructions

Add remaining 1 tablespoon oil to same skillet; heat over medium-high heat.

Add beaten eggs and cook until eggs are just set in center, tilting skillet and lifting edges of omelet with spatula to let uncooked portion flow underneath, about 3 minutes.

Top with fennel mixture. Sprinkle dill over.

Using spatula, fold uncovered half of omelet over; slide onto plate.

Garnish with chopped fennel and serve.

⬜

26. Outstanding Veggie Omelet

Ingredients
3 eggs, beaten
1 carrot, matchstick cut
3 scallions, diagonal sliced
1 handful tiny broccoli florets or whatever leftover veggies you have
Bits of leftover cooked turkey
Safflower oil
Low sodium salt

Instructions
Heat oil in a wok or large cast iron skillet over medium heat, until hot enough to sizzle a drop of water.
Add broccoli and carrots, stir fry 2 min. until soft.
Add cooked turkey, stir fry 1 min. until heated through. Add scallions and eggs, scramble. Add salt to taste.
Serve.
⸮

27. Basil Turkey with Roasted Tomatoes

Ingredients
2 turkey breasts
1 cup mushrooms, chopped
1/2 medium onion, chopped
1-2 tbsp extra virgin olive oil
Half cup thinly sliced fresh basil
low sodium salt and pepper, to taste
1 pint cherry tomatoes
Stevia to taste
Fresh parsley, for garnish

Instructions
Preheat the oven to 400 degrees F. Place the tomatoes on a baking sheet and drizzle with olive oil and stevia. Sprinkle with low sodium salt and pepper and toss to coat evenly. Bake for 15-20 minutes until soft. While the tomatoes are roasting, heat one tablespoon of olive oil in a large pan over low heat. Add the onions and mushrooms and cook for 10-12 minutes to soften and caramelize, stirring regularly. Clear a space for the chicken.

Season the turkey with low sodium salt and pepper and then place it in the pan. Simmer for 15 minutes or until the chicken is cooked through. Every 5 minutes or so, spoon the sauce in the pan over the turkey.

To assemble, divide the tomatoes between two plates. Place one turkey breast on each and then spoon the onions, mushrooms, and pan drippings over the turkey. Garnish with parsley.

⁇

28. Creamy Chicken Casserole

Ingredients
2 cups cubed cooked chicken
1 1/2 cups cooked butternut squash
1/2 cup coconut cream,
1/4 cup coconut oil, melted
1 heaping cup green peas, fresh or frozen
1 tbsp apple cider vinegar
1/2 tsp low sodium salt
1/2 tsp oregano
1/2 tsp thyme
1 tbsp fresh parsley

Instructions
In a large bowl, mash the butternut squash. Stir in the coconut cream, oil, vinegar, low sodium salt, oregano, and thyme.
Once everything is combined, add in chicken and peas.
Place the mixture into a large saucepan and cook over medium heat for 5-8 minutes.
Top with fresh parsley and serve warm.
⁇

29.   Spectacular Spaghetti and Delish Turkey Balls

Ingredients
1 spaghetti squash
Extra virgin olive oil,
low sodium salt and pepper
1 tsp dried or fresh oregano

For the sauce:
1 lb ground turkey
1 small onion, chopped
4 cloves garlic, minced
1 tbsp coconut oil
1 tomato, chopped
1/2 jar of tomato sauce
1 tbsp Italian seasoning
low sodium salt and pepper to taste
Fresh basil

Instructions
Preheat oven to 400 degrees F. Using a sharp knife, cut the squash in half lengthwise. Scoop out the seeds and discard.
Place the halves with the cut side up on a rimmed baking sheet. Drizzle with olive oil and season with low sodium salt, pepper, and oregano. Roast the squash in the oven for 40-45 minutes, until you can poke the squash easily with a fork.
Let it cool until you can handle it safely. Then scrape the insides with a fork to shred the squash into strands.
While the spaghetti squash is roasting, melt coconut oil in a large skillet over medium heat.
Add chopped onion and garlic and cook for 4-5 minutes. Add ground turkey and brown the meat, stirring occasionally. Season with low sodium salt and pepper.
Add the chopped tomato, tomato sauce, and Italian seasoning and stir to combine. Simmer on low heat, stirring occasionally, while the spaghetti squash finishes roasting. Serve over spaghetti squash with basil for garnish.
[?]

30.   Sensational Courgette Pasta and Turkey Bolognaise

Ingredients
4 medium zucchini
For the sauce:
1 lb ground turkey
1 small onion, chopped
4 cloves garlic, minced
1 tbsp coconut oil
1 tomato, chopped
1/2 jar of tomato sauce
1 tbsp Italian seasoning
low sodium salt and pepper to taste
Fresh basil, for garnish

Instructions
Use a julienne peeler to slice the zucchini into noodles, stopping when you reach the seeds. Set aside.
If cooking zucchini noodles, simply add to a skillet and sauté over medium heat for 4-5 minutes.
Melt coconut oil in a large skillet over medium heat. Add chopped onion and garlic and cook for 4-5 minutes.
Add ground turkey and brown the meat, stirring occasionally. Season with low sodium salt and pepper.
Add the chopped tomato, tomato sauce, and Italian seasoning and stir to combine. Simmer on low heat, stirring occasionally.
Add the sauce to the noodles and ENJOY.
⁂

31.   Sublime Courgette Tomato Salad

Ingredients
2 medium zucchini
2 tomatoes
cooking spray
low sodium salt
freshly ground black pepper
a few sprigs fresh parsley

Instructions
Heat your grill to high flame.
Wash zucchini and trim off the ends. Using a mandolin or vegetable peeler slice the zucchini lengthwise in thin slices.
Lightly spray with cooking spray and season with low sodium salt and pepper, to taste. Grill the zucchini ribbons on 1 side, until lightly marked and wilted, about 1 to 2 minutes. Remove and put on a platter and let cool slightly.
Cut up tomatoes in large chunks, season with low sodium salt and pepper to taste. Arrange on a platter with zucchini and garnish with parsley sprigs.
⏎

32.   Brussels Muscles Sprouts

Ingredients
6 oz Brussels sprouts, washed
2 tbsp olive oil
juice of 1 large lemon
low sodium salt and fresh cracked pepper, to taste

Instructions
With a large sharp knife, trim off the stems, cut the Brussels in half lengthwise, then place cut side down on the board and finely shred the sprouts.
Place in a large bowl and toss with olive oil, lemon juice, low sodium salt and pepper to taste.
▢

33.   Blushing Beet Salad

Ingredients
2 large beets, washed and stems cut off
1 cup carrots, peeled and cooked
1 tbsp cilantro, chopped
1 tbsp diced onion
2 tbsp paleo mayonnaise
Low sodium salt and pepper

Instructions
Boil beets in water until soft, about 50 minutes.
Peel and cut into small 1/2" cubes.
Cook carrots until tender and cut into bite size cubes.
Combine diced onion, carrots, beets, mayonnaise, cilantro, low sodium salt and pepper.
⁂

34. Sashimi Divine with Vinaigrette

Ingredients
5 oz sashimi tuna (sushi grade)
1 tsp extra virgin olive oil
1 tsp fresh lemon juice
2 cups baby arugula
1 tsp capers
Low sodium salt and fresh pepper

Instructions
Season tuna with low sodium salt and fresh cracked pepper.
Place arugula and capers on a plate. Combine oil and lemon juice, low sodium salt and pepper.
Heat your grill to high heat and clean grate well. When grill is hot, spray grate with oil to prevent sticking then place tuna on the grill; cook one minute without moving. Turnover and cook an additional minute; remove from heat and set aside on a plate.
Slice tuna on the diagonal and place on top of salad. Top with lemon vinaigrette and eat immediately.
⁇

35.　Grilled Shrimp Fennel Salad

Ingredients
1 lb jumbo shrimp, peeled and deveined (weight after peeled)
4 cups fresh arugula or baby greens
1 cup (1/2 small bulb) fresh fennel, thinly sliced or shaved w/ mandoline
1 medium-size ripe Hass avocado, sliced thin
For the vinaigrette:
3 tbsp fresh lemon juice
1 tbsp extra-virgin olive oil
3 tbsp minced shallots
 Low sodium salt, to taste
freshly ground black pepper, to taste

Instructions
For the vinaigrette:
Combine the lemon juice, olive oil, shallots, low sodium salt and pepper in a container with a tight-fitting lid and shake it vigorously to combine.
Reserve 1/2 cup of the vinaigrette for dressing the salad and pour the remaining vinaigrette into a medium nonreactive bowl. Put the shrimp in the bowl, season with low sodium salt and pepper and toss; let it sit for about 30 minutes.
Prepare your outdoor grill, or heat a grill pan over medium-high heat. Grill the shrimp until just cooked through and opaque, about 1 1/2 minutes per side. Transfer to a plate.
Divide the baby greens on four plates, top with sliced fennel, oranges, avocados and shrimp. Season with low sodium salt and pepper to taste and drizzle with the remaining vinaigrette, about 2 tbsp per salad.
⬚

36.   Chicken Delish Salad

Ingredients
1 lb skinless boneless chicken breast, cut into 1 inch cubes

For the marinade:
2 tbsp fresh squeezed lemon juice
1 tsp dried oregano
1 tsp garlic, crushed
Low sodium salt to taste
fresh ground black pepper to taste

For the salad:
1 1/4 cups cucumber, peeled
1 1/4 cups diced tomato
1/4 cup diced bell pepper
2 tbsp red onion, diced
1 1/2 tsp vinegar
1 1/2 tsp fresh lemon juice
2 tsp olive oil
1 tsp fresh parsley
1/8 tsp dried oregano
Low sodium salt and black pepper to taste
4 cups shredded lettuce
lemon wedges for serving

Instructions
Marinate the chicken at least 2-3 hours or overnight. If using wooden skewers, soak in water at least 30 minutes if grilling outdoors.
Combine the first 12 salad ingredients (cucumbers through low sodium salt and black pepper, not the lettuce) and set aside in the refrigerator to let the flavours set.
Thread chicken on 4 skewers and cook on a hot grill (indoor or outdoor grill) until chicken is cooked through, about 10-12 minutes.
Divide lettuce between four plates, top with tomato-cucumber salad, and grilled chicken. Serve with lemon wedges.
⁇

37. Ostrich Steak or Venison with Divine Mustard Sauce and Roasted Tomatoes

Ingredients
For the tomatoes:
2 pints cherry tomatoes, halved
2 tbsp extra virgin olive oil
Stevia to taste
low sodium salt and freshly ground pepper

For the cauliflower rice:
1/2 head of cauliflower, chopped coarsely
1/2 small onion, finely diced
1 tbsp coconut oil
1 tbsp fresh parsley, chopped
low sodium salt and freshly ground pepper, to taste

For the meat:
4 Ostrich or venison steaks
Extra virgin olive oil
low sodium salt and freshly ground pepper
Coconut oil, for the pan

For the sauce:
1/4 cup red onion, finely diced
1/4 cup apple cider vinegar
1 cup low sodium chicken stock
1 tbsp whole grain mustard
low sodium salt and freshly ground pepper, to taste

Instructions
Preheat the oven to 400 degrees F. Place the tomatoes on a baking sheet and drizzle with olive oil and honey. Sprinkle with low sodium salt and pepper and toss to coat evenly. Bake for 15-20 minutes until soft.
While the tomatoes are roasting, prepare the cauliflower rice. Place the cauliflower into a food processor and pulse until reduced to the size of rice grains.

Melt the coconut oil in a nonstick skillet over medium heat. Add the onion and cook for 5-6 minutes until translucent. Stir in the cauliflower, season with low sodium salt and pepper, and cover. Cook for 7-10 minutes until the cauliflower has softened, and then toss with parsley.

To make the lamb, preheat the oven to 325 degrees F. Pat the ostrich or venison dry and rub with olive oil. Generously season both sides with low sodium salt and pepper.

Heat one tablespoon of coconut oil in a cast iron skillet. When the pan is hot, add to the pan and sear for 2-3 minutes on all sides until golden brown.

Place the skillet in the oven and bake for 5-8 minutes until the ostrich or venison reaches desired doneness. Let rest for 10 minutes before serving.

While the meat is resting, add the red onion to the skillet with the pan drippings from the lamb. Sauté for 3-4 minutes, then add the white wine vinegar.

Turn the heat to high and cook until the vinegar has mostly evaporated. Add the stock and bring to a boil, cooking until the sauce reduces by half.

Stir in the mustard, and season to taste with low sodium salt and pepper. Pour over ostrich or venison to serve.

☐

38.   Tantalizing Turkey Pepper Stir-fry

Ingredients
2 bell peppers, sliced
1 cup broccoli florets
2 cooked and shredded turkey breasts
1/4 teaspoon chili powder
low sodium salt and pepper to taste
1 tablespoon coconut oil for frying

Instructions
Add 1 tablespoon coconut oil into a frying pan on a medium heat.
Place the sliced bell peppers into the frying pan.
After the bell peppers soften, add in the cooked turkey meat.
Add in the chili powder, low sodium salt and pepper.
Mix well and stir-fry for a few more minutes.
?

39.   Cheeky Chicken Stir Fry

Ingredients

1 pound boneless, skinless chicken breast

2 tablespoons coconut oil

1 medium onion, finely chopped (about 1 cup)

2 heads broccoli, sliced into 3-inch spears (about 4 cups)

2 medium carrots, sliced (about 1 cup)

2 heads baby bok choy, sliced crosswise into 1-inch strips (about 1½ cups)

4 ounces shiitake mushrooms, stemmed and thinly sliced (about 1 cup)

1 small zucchini, sliced (about 1 cup)

½ teaspoon low sodium salt

Garlic powder to taste

1½ cups water

Instructions

Rinse the chicken and pat dry. Cut into 1-inch cubes and transfer to a plate.

Heat the coconut oil in a large skillet over medium heat

Saute the onion for 8 to 10 minutes, until soft and translucent

Add the broccoli, carrots, and chicken and saute for 10 minutes until almost tender

Add the bok choy, mushrooms, zucchini, and low sodium salt and saute for 5 minutes

Add 1 cup of the water, cover the skillet, and cook for about 10 minutes, until the vegetables are wilted

In a small bowl, dissolve the arrowroot powder in the remaining ½ cup of water, stirring until thoroughly combined

Season at the end with garlic powder, salt and if you like some chilli powder

⏺

40.   Chicken Fennel Stir-Fry

Ingredients
3 chicken breasts or the meat from 1 whole roasted chicken
2 tablespoons coconut oil
1 onion
1 bulb of fennel
1 teaspoon each of low sodium salt, pepper, garlic powder and basil

Instructions
Stovetop:
Cut the chicken into bite sized pieces. If chicken is raw, heat butter/coconut oil in large skillet or wok until melted.
Add chicken and cook on medium/high heat until chicken is cooked through. (If chicken is pre-cooked, cook the vegetables first then add chicken)
While cooking, cut the onion into bite sized pieces (1/2 inch) and thinly slice the fennel bulb into thin slivers.
Add all to skillet or wok, add spices and continue sautéing until all are cooked through and fragrant.
This will take approximately 10-12 minutes.

41. Moroccan Madness

Ingredients
1 chicken breast, chopped into pieces
1/2 tbsp olive oil
1/2 onion, chopped
1 bell pepper, chopped
1 cup diced courgette
2 cloves garlic, minced
1 tsp ginger, minced
1 tsp cumin
1 tsp turmeric
1/2 tsp paprika
1/2 tbsp oregano
1/2 can diced tomatoes
1/2 cup low sodium chicken stock
low sodium salt and pepper

Instructions
In a pan cook the chicken in the olive oil
Once it's finished cooking, remove from pan and set aside
Add to the pan the bell pepper, onion, courgette, garlic, ginger and all spices, sauté until bell pepper and onion become soft
Add back in the chicken along with the diced tomatoes and chicken stock, let simmer for 1o minutes
⁂

42.   Golden Glazed Drumsticks

Ingredients
8 medium chicken drumsticks, skin removed
olive oil spray 1 cup water
1/3 cup rice vinegar
1/3 cup low sodium gluten free soy sauce
4 drops stevia
3 cloves garlic, crushed
1 tsp ginger, grated
2 tbsp chives or scallions, chopped
1 tsp sesame seeds

Instructions
In a heavy large saucepan, brown chicken on high for 3-4 minutes with a little spray oil. Add water, vinegar, soy sauce, stevia, garlic, ginger and cook on high until liquid comes to a boil.
Reduce heat to low and simmer, covered for about 20 minutes.
Remove cover and bring heat to high, allowing sauce to reduce down, about 8-10 minutes, until it becomes thick, turning chicken occasionally. (Keep an eye on glaze, you don't want it to burn when it starts becoming thick) Transfer chicken to a platter and pour sauce on top.
Top with chives and sesame seeds and serve.
?

43.　Piquant Peanut Chicken

Ingredients
3/4 cup green onion, chopped
1 1/4 cups shredded carrots
1 1/4 cups cup shredded broccoli slaw
1 cup bean sprouts
2 tbsp chopped salt free peanuts
1 lime, sliced
cilantro for garnish (optional)
For the Peanut Sauce:
14.5 oz fat free chicken broth
5 tbsp peanut butter
Stevia to taste
2 tbsp soy sauce (use Tamari for gluten free)
1 tbsp freshly grated ginger
2 cloves garlic, minced
For the chicken:
16 oz chicken breast, cut into thin strips
Low sodium salt and pepper (to taste)
1 tspn chilli flakes
juice of 1/2 lime
5 cloves garlic, crushed
1 tbsp fresh ginger, grated
1 tbsp soy sauce (use Tamari for gluten free)
1/2 tbsp sesame oil

Instructions
For the peanut sauce:
Combine 1 cup chicken broth, peanut butter, stevia, 2 tbsp soy sauce, ginger, and 3 cloves crushed garlic in a small saucepan and simmer over medium-low heat stirring occasionally until sauce becomes smooth and well blended, about 5-10 minutes. Set aside.
Season chicken with low sodium salt and pepper, chilli, lime, garlic, ginger and soy sauce.
Heat a large skillet or wok until hot. Add oil and sauté chicken on high heat until cooked through, about 2-3 minutes; remove from heat and set aside. Add 2 cloves crushed garlic, scallions, carrots, broccoli slaw and/or bean sprouts and low sodium salt, sauté until tender crisp, about 1-2 minutes. Divide chicken

between 6 bowls, top with sauteed vegetables, bean sprouts, chopped peanuts (or you can toss everything together to hide the vegetables so your family members don't push them aside!) and garnish with cilantro and lime wedges.

⁂

44.   Cheeky Chicken Salad

Ingredients
olive oil spray
2 tsp olive oil
16 oz (2 large) skinless boneless chicken breasts, cut into 24 1-inch chunks
Low sodium salt and pepper to taste
4 cups shredded romaine
1 cup shredded red cabbage

For the Skinny Cheeky Sauce:
2 1/2 tbsppaleo mayonnaise
2 tbsp scallions, chopped fine plus more for topping
1 1/2 tsp chilli flakes

Instructions
Preheat oven to 425°F. Spray a baking sheet with olive oil spray.
Season chicken with low sodium salt and pepper, olive oil and mix well so the olive oil evenly coats all of the chicken.
Meanwhile combine the sauce in a medium bowl. When the chicken is ready, drizzle it over the top and enjoy!!

⁂

45.   Melting Mustard Chicken

Ingredients
8 small chicken thighs, skin removed
3 tsp mustard powder
1 tbsppaleo mayonnaise
1 clove garlic, crushed
1 lime, squeezed, and lime zest
3/4 tsp pepper
Low sodium salt
dried parsley

Instructions
Preheat oven to 400°. Rinse the chicken and remove the skin and all fat. Pat dry …place in a large bowl and season generously with low sodium salt. In a small bowl combine mustard, mayonnaise, lime juice, lime zest, garlic and pepper. Mix well. Pour over chicken, tossing well to coat.
Spray a large baking pan with a little Pam to prevent sticking since all the fat and skin was removed from chicken. Place chicken to fit in a single layer.
Top the chicken with dried parsley. Bake until cooked through, about 30-35 minutes.
Finish the chicken under the broiler until it is golden brown. Serve chicken with the pan juices drizzled over the top.
⏹

46.   Tantalizing Turkey with Roasted Vegetables

Ingredients
10 (20 oz) Turkey Breasts
20 medium asparagus, ends trimmed, cut in half
3 red bell peppers
1 cup carrots, sliced in half long way
2 red onions, chopped in large chunks
10 oz sliced mushrooms
1/2 cup plus 2 tbsp rice vinegar
1/4 cup extra virgin olive oil
1 tsp stevia
Low sodium salt and pepper
3 tbsp fresh rosemary
2 cloves garlic, smashed and sliced
2 tbsp oregano or thyme
4 leaves fresh sage, chopped

Instructions
Preheat oven to 425°. Wash and dry the chicken well with a paper towel. Combine all the ingredients together and using your hands and arrange in a very large roasting pan.
The vegetables should not touch the turkey or it will steam instead of roast.
All ingredients should be spread out in a single layer. If necessary, use two baking sheets or disposable tins to achieve this. Bake for 35 - 40 minutes.
⁇

47.   Grilled Ostrich Steak

Ingredients
6 medium ostrich steaks
1 tbsp vinegar
garlic powder
black pepper ground to taste
oregano
2 tablespoons olive oil

Instructions
Season ostrich with vinegar and olive oil.
Add garlic powder, oregano and mix well....marinate at least 20 minutes.
Broil or grill on low until ostrich is cooked through, careful not to burn. Enjoy with green salad.
⍰

48.   Lemony Chicken and Asparagus

Ingredients
1 1/2 pounds skinless chicken breast, cut into 1-inch cubes
Low sodium salt, to taste
1/2 cup reduced-sodium chicken broth
2 tablespoons reduced-sodium soy sauce (or Tamari for GF)
2 tablespoons water
1 tbsp olive oil, divided
1 bunch asparagus, ends trimmed, cut into 2-inch pieces
6 cloves garlic, chopped
1 tbsp fresh ginger
3 tablespoons fresh lemon juice
fresh black pepper, to taste

Instructions
Lightly season the chicken with low sodium salt. In a small bowl, combine chicken broth and soy sauce. In a second small bowl combine the cornstarch and water and mix well to combine.
Heat a large non-stick wok over medium-high heat, when hot add 1 teaspoon of the oil, then add the asparagus and cook until tender-crisp, about 3 to 4 minutes. Add the garlic and ginger and cook until golden, about 1 minute. Set aside.
Increase the heat to high, then add 1 teaspoon of oil and half of the chicken and cook until browned and cooked through, about 4 minutes on each side. Remove and set aside and repeat with the remaining oil and chicken. Set aside.
Add the soy sauce mixture; bring to a boil and cook about 1-1/2 minutes. Add lemon juice and stir well, when it simmers return the chicken and asparagus to the wok and mix well, remove from heat and serve.
⬚

49.   Easy Paleo Spaghetti Squash & Meatballs

Ingredients

One medium spaghetti squash.

One pound of ground Italian sausage.

One can of tomato sauce, I used a 14 ounce can.

2 tbsp of hot pepper relish (optional).

4 to 6 cloves of garlic, whole.

2 tbsp of olive oil.

Italian seasoning (Oregano, Basil, Thyme) to taste, I used about 2 tsp

Instruction

Make sure you use a large 6 quart slow cooker for this recipe.

Dump your tomato sauce, olive oil, garlic, hot pepper relish and Italian seasoning into your slow cooker and stir well.

Cut your squash in half and scoop out the seeds.

Place your 2 squash halves face down into your slow cooker.

Roll your ground sausage into meatballs, then fit as many as you can in the sauce around the squash. I was able to work in about a half pound worth.

Cook on High for 3 hours or cook on low for 5 hours.

Use a large fork to pull the "spaghetti" out of your squash, then top with your meatballs and sauce.

Garnish with parsley if you feel fancy, and enjoy!

⬜

50.   Meatball Zucchini Skillet

Ingredients
Grass-fed butter (coconut oil would also work but the butter gives a great flavour)
1/2 large vidalia onion
1 pound grass-fed ground beef (if using lean beef you may need to add an egg to hold the meatballs together)
1 1/2 tsp garlic powder
1 1/2 tsp onion powder
1 tsp Italian seasoning
2 medium zucchinis
2 medium tomatoes
sea salt and pepper to taste

Instructions
Put your skillet on medium-high heat.
Then dice your onions and add them to the skillet with 1-2 tbsp of butter. Saute for around 5 minutes until translucent.
While the onions are cooking take your grass-fed ground beef and roll them into small 1 1/2 inch balls (we came up with about 20). Add the meatballs to the pan and cook for around 10 minutes, stirring them occasionally, flipping them over to get even cooking, and adding any additional butter if needed to prevent sticking (<< we didn't need any since our beef had a higher fat content, but if you are using lean ground beef the extra butter may be necessary).
When the beef is cooking wash and dice up the zucchini and tomatoes. Add those to the skillet next along with the seasonings.
Place a lid over the skillet and reduce to medium heat. Cook for around 5 minutes then remove the lid, stir and put it back on top of the skillet. We cooked the beef and vegetables for another 5 minutes or so until tender, but keep checking them to see when they are done for you.
Finally plate up some of the meatballs and vegetables topping with salt and pepper as desired.
⁊

51.   Finger Lickin' Chipotle Meatballs

Ingredients

1 large, deep frying pan

1 large brown onion, peeled and diced finely

1 tsp of lard or ghee (clarified butter)

For the meatballs mix

800g of grass fed beef mince (1.8 pounds ground beef)

3 medium dried chipotle chilies (tinned chipotle can also be used), seeds out

2 tbsp chopped fresh coriander (cilantro)

2 large garlic cloves, finely diced

1 tsp ground coriander seed or powder

1 tsp ground cumin seed or powder

1 tsp sweet or medium paprika

1 tbsp virgin olive oil

1 ½ tsp of sea salt

2 tbsp lard (I used a mix of lard and ghee)

For the sauce

½ of the onion mentioned above

2 garlic cloves, finely chopped

2 medium chipotle chilies, seeds out

½ tsp ground coriander seed or powder

1 tsp ground cumin seed or powder

½ tsp paprika

2 bay leaves

400g of diced tomatoes or tomato puree (about 1 ½ cups)

½ tsp sea salt

Instructions

If using dried chipotle chilies, place in hot water for at least an hour before using to rehydrate.

Sauté the onion in lard or ghee for 3-5 minutes, until translucent. Use half of the onion in the meatball mix and reserve the rest for the sauce.

While onion is cooking, pre-chop other ingredients for the meatballs. Slice the chipotle chilies in half and remove the seeds. Chop or grind with mortar and pestle.

Combine beef mince with half of the cooked onion, chopped garlic, chipotle chilies, paprika, cumin, coriander seed, salt and olive oil. Combine and knead with your hands. Using clean, wet hands roll the mix into small balls (somewhere between a walnut and a golf ball size). Set aside until ready to cook.
Preheat a dollop of lard in the large frying pan until sizzling hot. Cook the meatballs on medium/high heat for 3 minutes on each side, until well browned.
Add the rest of the cooked onion, garlic, two chopped chilies and sauce spices to the pan with the meatballs. Stir through and add the tomato puree. Combine and cook for 8-10 minutes uncovered, stirring frequently to make sure the meatballs cook evenly and the sauce is well combined. Taste for salt. Drizzle with a little lime juice before serving.

Preparation time: 20 minutes
Cooking time: 20 minutes

52. Vegetarian Curry with Squash

Ingredients

1 tbsp coconut oil

2 cups mixed raw nuts.

1 medium yellow onion, diced

1 tsp low sodium salt

1 green bell pepper, thinly sliced

4 cloves garlic, minced

1-inch piece fresh ginger, peeled and minced

1 14-oz. can coconut milk

1 large acorn squash, peeled, seeded, and cut into 1-inch cubes

2 tsp lime juice

One teaspoon curry powder (mild or hot)

1/4 cup cilantro, chopped

Cauliflower rice, for serving

Instructions

Melt the coconut oil in a large pan over medium heat. Add the onion and cook for 5-6 minutes, stirring occasionally. Add the bell pepper, garlic, ginger, and low sodium salt and stir to combine. Cook for an additional minute.

Add the curry powder to the pan and cook for about a minute, stirring to coat the other ingredients. Add in the coconut milk and bring to a simmer. Stir in the squash.

Simmer, stirring occasionally, for 15-20 minutes until the squash is fork-tender. Remove the pan from the heat and stir in the lime juice. Taste and adjust low sodium salt and lime juice as necessary. Sprinkle with cilantro to serve.

Roast the nuts under the grill until crisp and sprinkle over the top of the curry.

[?]

53.   Rucola Salad

Ingredients
4 teaspoons fresh lemon juice
4 teaspoons walnut oil
low sodium salt and freshly ground pepper
6 cups rucola leaves and tender stems (about 6 ounces)
Garlic powder to taste

Instructions
Pour the lemon juice into a large bowl. Gradually whisk in the oil. Season with low sodium salt and pepper. Add the greens, toss until evenly dressed and serve at once. This is delicious, and feel free to add tomatoes or grated carrot and onion slices.
Substitution: Any mild green, such as lamb's lettuce will do.
⏧

54.   Tasty Spring Salad

Ingredients
5 cups of any salad greens in season of your choice
Dressing:
125 mL (1/2 cup) olive oil
45 mL (3 tbsp) lemon juice
15 mL (1 tbsp) pure mustard powder
45 mL (3 tbsp) capers, minced (optional)
low sodium salt
pepper

Instructions
Combine salad greens and any other raw vegetables of choice.
Combine oil, lemon juice and mustard. Mix well.
Add capers, low sodium salt and pepper to taste.
Pour dressing over salad, toss and serve.
⏧

55.   Spinach and Dandelion Pomegranate Salad

Ingredients
1 small bunch fresh spinach
12 dandelion leaves
1 cup pomegranate seeds
1/2 cup pecan halves

Instructions
You may substitute appropriate fresh greens for the dandelion and sorrel leaves.
Wash and destem spinach. Pick and wash sorrel and dandelions.
Coarsely chop dandelion leaves, and tear spinach, then toss dandelion, sorrel and spinach together in a stainless steel bowl.
Put aside in refrigerator to drain and cool.
When drained, pour off excess water, and add pomegranate and pecans. Toss with dressing and serve.
🞂

56.   Delicious Chicken Salad

Ingredients
Cooked and chopped chicken breast
Chopped almonds
Mashed avocado
Lots of low sodium salt and pepper
Any lettuce leaves of choice

Instructions
Mix the first six ingredients together in a bowl, season with low sodium salt and pepper, and then spoon onto lettuce leaves.
Roll up and enjoy!
🞂

57. Avocado Tuna Salad

Ingredients
2 tins high quality albacore tuna
1 avocado
1/4 of an onion, chopped
juice of 1/2 a lime
2 Tbsp cilantro (or sub basil if you prefer)
some low sodium salt and pepper, to taste

Instructions
Shred the tuna.
Add all of the other ingredients and mix.
⬚

58. Macadamia Nut Chicken/Turkey Salad

Ingredients
1lb chicken/turkey breast
1tsp macadamia nut oil, or oil of choice
few pinches of low sodium salt and pepper
1/2 cup macadamia nuts, chopped
1/2 cup diced celery
3 tbsp divine dressing
2 tbsp julienned basil
1 tbsp lemon juice

Instructions
Preheat oven to 350. Place chicken breasts on sheet tray, drizzle will oil and a pinch of low sodium salt and pepper.
 Bake for about 35 minutes until cooked through. Remove from oven and let cool.
In a large bowl shred chicken. Add nuts, celery, basil, mayo, lemon juice, and a pinch of low sodium salt and pepper. Gently stir until combined. Eat!
Divine Dressing:
Mix together, 4 Tbsp. chili powder, 1 tsp each garlic powder, onion powder, and oregano, 2 tsp each paprika and cumin, 4 tsp low sodium salt, and 1/8-1/4 tsp red pepper flakes. Add 1 cup olive oil and half cup rice vinegar.

?

59.   Red Cabbage Bonanza Salad

Ingredients
For the chicken or turkey:
450g chicken/turkey mince, free range of course
1 long red chili, finely chopped with the seeds
2 garlic cloves, finely chopped
Little nob of fresh ginger, peeled and finely chopped
1 stem lemon grass, pale section only, finely chopped
1/2 bunch of coriander stems washed and finely chopped (I don't waste anything, save the leaves for the salad)
1 tbsp low sodium salt
1 tbsp coconut aminos
1/2 lime rind grated
1/2 lime, juiced
A pinch of low sodium salt
Coconut oil for frying (about 3 tablespoons)

For the salad:
1/4 red cabbage, thinly sliced
1 large carrot, peeled and grated
1/2 Spanish onion, thinly sliced
2 tbsps green spring onion, chopped
1/2 bunch of fresh coriander leaves (saved from the stems used in the chicken)
A handful of fresh mint or Thai basil if available
1/2 cup crashed roasted cashews or some sesame seeds
1/2 cup dried fried shallots (optional for garnish)
2 tbsp toasted coconut flakes (optional for garnish)

For the dressing:
2 tbsp olive oil
3 tbsps lime juice
1 small red chili, finely chopped (you can leave it out if you like it mild)

Instructions
Once you've prepared all your ingredients for the chicken, heat 1 tbsp of coconut oil in a large frying pan or a wok to high. Throw in lemongrass, chili, garlic, coriander stems and ginger and stir fry for about a minute until fragrant.

Add chicken mince and lime zest. Stir and break apart the mince with a wooden mixing spoon until separated into small

The meat will now be changing to white colour. Add lime juice. Stir through and cook for a further few minutes. Total cooking time for the chicken should be about 10 minutes.

Prepare the salad base by mixing together sliced red cabbage, onion grated carrot, and fresh herbs.

Mix all dressing ingredients and toss through the salad.

Serve cooked chicken mince on top of the dressed salad and topped with roasted cashews, dried shallots, coconut flakes and extra fresh herbs.

⁇

60. Spectacular Sprouts Salad

Ingredients
1/2 pound of mixed sprouts (2-ish cups once sliced)
1/2 Granny Smith apple
1/2 cup chopped almonds
2 chicken breasts, chopped
1/2 white onion, finely diced

Vinaigrette:
2 TBSP Apple Cider Vinegar
1 TBSP quality brown mustard
1 TBSP avocado oil
Stevia to taste
1/2 tsp low sodium salt
few grinds of black pepper

Instructions
Cut Granny Smith apple, slicing into matchsticks.
Chop the half cup of almonds. Finely dice the white onion. Scallions would work too if you prefer a more mild onion flavour... though the white did not overpower.
Remove the breasts and chop into bite-sized pieces. Combine all of these ingredients into a large bowl and gently toss the sprouts into the salad.
Whipping up the vinaigrette takes seconds. Add all ingredients to a small bowl and whisk until smooth.
Pour over the sprouts salad and toss to bring together.
⏺

61.   Avocado Egg Salad

Ingredients
Cooked and chopped organic eggs x 3
Chopped almonds
Mashed avocado
low sodium salt and pepper
Any lettuce leaves

Instructions
Mix the ingredients together in a bowl, season with low sodium salt and pepper, and then spoon onto lettuce leaves. Roll up and enjoy!
⬚

62.   Avocado Divine Salad

Ingredients
1 kilo boneless, skinless chicken or turkey breasts (2 or 3)
1 avocado
1/4 of an onion, chopped
juice of one lime and one lemon
2 tbsps cilantro (or sub basil if you prefer)
some low sodium salt and pepper, to taste
One bag mixed lettuce leaves
One tablespoon olive oil

Instructions
Cook chicken breast until done, let cool, and then shred. Add all of the other ingredients and mix.
⬚

63.　Classic Waldorf Salad

Ingredients
half whole cooked chicken or turkey (~2lbs)
half cup apple, peeled and chopped (optional)
half cup onion, chopped (I like red, scallions are also good)
2-3 stalks celery, chopped (or .5 cup)
half cup pecans, chopped (optional)
half tsp low sodium salt
half tsp Lemon Garlic
pepper
1 tbsp lemon juice

Divine Dressing:
Mix together, 4 Tbsp. chili powder, 1 tsp each garlic powder, onion powder, and oregano, 2 tsp each paprika and cumin, 4 tsp low sodium salt, and 1/8-1/4 tsp red pepper flakes. Add 1 cup olive oil and half cup rice vinegar

Instructions
First cook up a whole chicken. You can buy a rotisserie chicken, or do what I do, throw a chicken in the crockpot, sprinkle it with cumin, low sodium salt & pepper and let it cook for about 4-6 hours on low.
After the chicken is cooked and cooled, de-bone and shred the meat (white and dark) and put it in a large mixing bowl. I usually use about half of my 3-4lb chicken.
Then do a bunch of chopping. Peel your apple, then chop your apple, onions, celery, and pecans.
Combine all of these ingredients in the bowl with your chicken and then start adding the dressing. You want enough to cover all the ingredients and make them moist, but not overly runny or dry.
Add the low sodium salt and pepper, and lemon juice Stir well to combine. Add dressing.
⬚

64. Classic Tuna Salad

Ingredients

2 large grilled tuna steaks

2 tablespoons olive oil

.5 cup onion, chopped (I like red, scallions are also good)

2-3 stalks celery, chopped (or .5 cup)

.5 – .75 cup pecans, chopped (optional)

.5 – 1 tsp low sodium salt

.5 tsp Lemon Garlic pepper

.5 – 1 Tbsp lemon juice

Instructions

Grill the tuna steaks medium rare with garlic powder and black pepper to taste

Then do a bunch of chopping. Onions, celery, and pecans.

Combine all of these ingredients in the bowl with your cubed tuna and then start adding the dressing of oil and lemon juice seasoned.

You want enough to cover all the ingredients and make them moist, but not overly runny or dry.

It tastes great served right away, but even better after it sits in the fridge for a day.

⏎

65.   Artichoke Tuna Delight

Ingredients
1.5 cups diced grilled tuna
¼ cup finely diced red onion
1 small carrot julienned and cut into small pieces (or ½ a diced red bell pepper)
4-5 artichoke hearts (I used canned in water) diced
2 tablespoons capers
low sodium salt and pepper to taste.
6 Radicchio leaves

Instructions
Place all ingredients, except the radicchio leaves in a large bowl and combine.
Place a scoop if salad into each Radicchio cup and serve.
Store salad in an air tight container in the fridge.
[?]

66.   Tasty Tuna Stuffed Tomato

Ingredients
2 large tomatoes
Lettuce leaves (optional)
 2 (5 or 6 oz.) cans wild albacore tuna
6 Tbsp. olive oil and 1 tablespoon rice vinegar
1 stalk celery, chopped
1/2 small onion, chopped
1/4 tsp. low sodium salt
1/4 tsp. ground black pepper

Instructions
Wash and dry the tomatoes and remove any stem. You can either slice off the top part of the tomatoes and hollow them out, or cut each tomato into wedges, making sure to only cut down to about 1/2 inch before you get to the bottom of the tomato.
Arrange the tomatoes on a plate on top of lettuce leaves (optional).
Combine the remaining ingredients in a mixing bowl and add additional low sodium salt and/or pepper if desired. Spoon into the tomatoes and serve.
⸮

67.   Mediterranean Medley Salad

Ingredients
1 roasted chicken (organic, soy-free and pastured is best).. or turkey or ostrich steak

Dressing:
1/2 cup of olive oil, ¼ cup applecider vinegar and garlic powder and chilli powder to taste
1/4 cup fresh cilantro, chopped
1 head of romaine or butter lettuce
1 red onion, diced
1 lemon, juiced
low sodium salt and pepper as desired

Instructions
Shred the chicken/turkey etc or chop up and put it in a big bowl.
Add the dressing...also red onion, cilantro, lemon, low sodium salt and pepper.

Mix well and serve on a lettuce boat.

[?]

68.   Paleo Crock Pot Cashew Chicken

Ingredients

1/4 cup arrowroot starch

1/2 tsp. black pepper

2 lbs. chicken thighs, cut into bite-size pieces

1 tbs. coconut oil

3 tbs. coconut aminos

2 tbs. rice wine vinegar

2 tbs. organic ketchup (tomato paste would work also)

1/2-1 tbs. palm sugar

2 minced garlic cloves

1/2 tsp. minced fresh ginger

1/4-1/2 red pepper flakes

1/2 cup raw cashews

Instructions

Place starch and black pepper in a large Ziploc bag. Add chicken pieces and seal; toss to thoroughly coat meat.

Melt coconut oil in a large skillet or wok. Add chicken and cook for about 5 minutes until brown on all sides. Remove and add to crock pot.

Mix coconut aminos through red pepper flakes in a small bowl. Pour mixture over chicken and toss to coat. Put lid on crock pot and cook on low for 3-4 hours.

Stir cashews into chicken and sauce before serving.

[?]

69.   Spicy Slow Cooker Chorizo Chili

Ingredients

1 pound of grass fed beef

2 fresh chorizo sausages, casings removed (about 1/2 pound)

1 onion, diced

1 teaspoon of minced garlic

1 15 oz can of tomato sauce

1 15 oz can of diced tomatoes

1 can of rotel, I used hot

2 chipotle peppers in adobo, chopped

2 Tablespoons of chili powder

1 Tablespoon of cumin

salt and pepper to taste

Instructions

brown off all the meat in a skillet

drain and toss in the crock pot

in the same skillet add onions and garlic and cook just long enough to get some colour on those onions

(you may skip this step and just toss it in the crock pot, but I just personally like to get some colour on the onions before adding them in)

toss remaining ingredients in the crock pot and stir together

cook on low for 6-8 hours or on high for 4-6 hours

top with diced avocado, minced red onion and cilantro to serve

?

70.   Paleo Pulled Pork Sliders

Ingredients
Large pork roast
1 large onion, sliced
3 minced garlic cloves
2 tsp cumin
2 tsp chili powder
1 tsp pepper
2 tsp oregano
1 tsp paprika
1/2 tsp cayenne pepper
1/2 tsp cinnamon
2 tsp sea salt
juice of 1 lime
juice of 1 lemon

Instructions
Stir together the spices and rub all over the roast. Lay the onion slices down on the bottom of the slow cooker, and squeeze half of the fruit juices in. Put the roast in the crockpot and squeeze the remaining lime and lemon juice over it. Cook on low overnight or throughout the day about 8 hours (you really can't overcook it to be honest). When done, shred it with two forks until it's completely 'pulled'.

The "Buns"
1 large sweet potato (try to go for a nice evenly round one, remember the diameter will be the size of your sliders)
2 tbsp coconut oil
1/4 tsp cumin
1/4 tsp paprika
dash of sea salt

Instructions
Slice the sweet potato into 1/4" thick rounds. Lay them out on a parchment paper-lined cookie sheet. Brush each slice with coconut oil and sprinkle with the spices, then flip and do the same on the other side. Bake at 425 degrees Farenheit for 35 minutes until golden brown on the outside and cooked all the way through, flipping halfway through. You may need to crank it up to 450 if your oven isn't nice and sizzly.

Top a patty with pulled pork, and add any other toppings or sauces you'd like (I just used some lettuce from our garden).

Finish with the top patty and enjoy your delightful little sliders!

⏹

71.   Crock-Pot Roast

Ingredients

4 lb (1816g) beef chuck roast

1 tbsp (14g) light oil (for sautéing … such as coconut, olive or ghee)

1 cup (232g) red wine, good quality

4 each (12g) garlic cloves

10 sprigs (10g) fresh thyme

1 each (.64g) bay leaf

1 large (72g) carrot, peeled and cut into chunks

2 each (101g) celery ribs, cut into chunks

1 small (110g) onion, cut into chunks

1 small (420g) head cauliflower, leaves removed and cut into florets

salt and fresh cracked pepper, to taste

Instructions

Turn on your slow cooker, setting it to low.

Season your beef with a good layer and salt and pepper.

Heat a large sauté pan or skillet over medium high heat. Add your oil to the pan and swirl it around. Quickly add your beef to the pan and sear it, until a nice brown crust has formed. Flip it over and sear the other side. Continue flipping it, until all sides have been properly seared. Add your beef to the crock pot. Pour your red wine into the still very hot pan, with all the "stuff" stuck to the bottom. This should QUICKLY boil, releasing some of those little flavour morsels into the hot wine. Swirl the pan around and use a wooden spoon to scrape anything else off the bottom of the pan, into the wine. Pour the wine mixture over the top of the beef.

Add your garlic, thyme and bay leaves to the slow cooker, making sure it's pushed into the liquid.

Add the rest of the vegetables, except the cauliflower. Season with a bit of salt and pepper. Again, push these into the areas on the side of the roast, as much as possible. You don't want much of it covering the roast. You want most of the veggies on the sides, surrounding the roast. As this all cooks, the meat and veggies will shrink, releasing their juices, creating an AMAZING flavour, as well as creating its own natural juices, in which to cook! Getting everything as close to the bottom of the pot, as is possible, will help this process along.

Add the lid and allow the ingredients to cook for 8 hours.

After 8 hours, add your cauliflower to the pot and push the florets under the surface of the liquid, as much as possible. Season with a bit of salt and pepper. Cover and allow to cook for 20 minutes. Serve!

⁂

72.   Paleo Mini Meatloaves

Ingredients

2 pounds ground meat – mixture of grass fed beef and/or pork and/or veal

10 ounces frozen, chopped spinach

1-2 teaspoons oil

1 medium onion, finely diced

6 ounces mushrooms, finely diced

2 carrots, grated or finely diced

4 eggs, lightly beaten

1/3 cup coconut flour

2 teaspoons salt

2 teaspoons pepper

2 teaspoons onion powder

1 teaspoon garlic powder

1 teaspoon dried thyme

1/4 teaspoon grated nutmeg

Instructions

Preheat oven to 375 degrees F

Thaw the spinach, squeeze out the excess water and set aside.

Heat a pan on medium heat, add the oil and fry the onions and mushrooms until the onions are translucent and some of the liquid has cooked out of the mushrooms. Set aside to cool.

Place the ground meat in a large bowl, add the spinach, carrots, mushroom/onion mixture, beaten eggs, coconut flour and all the spices. Use your hands to combine it well but do not overmix.

Fill 18 regular size muffin tins to the top with the meatloaf mixture. (Greasing the tins may be a good idea if the meat you're using is fairly lean)

Cook for 20-25 minutes or until internal temperature reaches 160 degrees.

Allow to cool and use a knife to loosen meatloaves from sides of the pan before removing.

[?]

73.   Eggplant Bolognese with Zucchini Noodles (Low Carb)

Ingredients
1 1/2 lbs. eggplant, diced
1/2 lb. ground beef
2 tbsp extra virgin olive oil
Salt and freshly ground pepper
1 large yellow onion, chopped
3 cloves garlic, minced
2 bay leaves
4 sprigs thyme
1 tbsp tomato paste
1/2 cup red wine
1 28-oz. can whole peeled plum tomatoes
6 leaves fresh basil, chiffonade

Instructions
Heat the olive oil in a large pan over medium-high heat. Add in the onion and beef and sprinkle with salt and pepper. Cook for 8-10 minutes until the meat is browned. Stir in the eggplant, garlic, bay leaves, and thyme and sauté for an additional 15 minutes.
Once the eggplant is tender, stir in the tomato paste. Add the wine and scrape any browned bits off the bottom of the pan. Stir in the tomatoes and slightly crush with a spoon. Bring the mixture to a boil, then reduce the heat and simmer for 10 minutes, stirring occasionally. Adjust salt to taste. Serve warm garnished with fresh basil.

Notes
Servings: 4-6
Difficulty: Medium
⬚

74. Melt In Your Mouth Slow Cooker Beef Brisket

Ingredients
2 lbs. beef brisket
1 large onion, chopped
6 carrots, diced
8 oz. mushrooms, sliced
6 cloves garlic, peeled and sliced
3 cups beef broth
4 fresh thyme sprigs
1/2 tsp salt
Freshly ground pepper

Instructions
Add the onion, carrots, mushrooms, and garlic to the slow cooker. Pour in the beef broth and then add the brisket. Sprinkle with salt and pepper and add the thyme. Cover and cook on low heat for 8-16 hours, until the meat is tender.

Notes
Servings: 4
Difficulty: Easy
⏤

75. Bacon-Wrapped Roasted Asparagus

Ingredients
1 bunch asparagus, ends trimmed
4 pieces bacon
Extra virgin olive oil
Salt and pepper, to taste
Maple syrup, optional

Instructions
Preheat the oven to 400 degrees F. Place the bacon in a large skillet. Cook for about 3 minutes per side, until the bacon gets just a little crisp. Remove to a paper towel-lined plate.
Line a rimmed baking sheet with aluminum foil or a Silpat. Wash and dry the asparagus and then place it on the baking sheet. Drizzle with olive oil and toss to coat. Sprinkle with salt and pepper.
Divide the asparagus into 4 small bundles. Wrap a piece of bacon around each bundle of asparagus and place on the baking sheet. Brush the bacon with maple syrup if desired. Bake for 10-12 minutes, or until the bacon is crisp. Serve immediately.

Notes
Servings: 4
Difficulty: Easy
⁇

76.   Simple Cod Piccata

Ingredients
1 lb. cod fillets
1/3 cup almond flour
1/2 tsp salt
2-3 tbsp extra virgin olive oil
2 tbsp grapeseed oil, divided
3/4 cup chicken stock
3 tbsp lemon juice
1/4 cup capers, drained
2 tbsp fresh parsley, chopped

Instructions
Stir the almond flour and salt together in a shallow bowl. Rinse off the fish and pat dry with a paper towel. Dredge the fish in the almond flour mixture to coat.
Heat enough olive oil to coat the bottom of a large skillet over medium-high heat along with one tablespoon grapeseed oil. Working in batches, add the cod and cook for 2-3 minutes per side to brown. Remove to a plate and set aside.
Add the chicken stock, lemon juice, and capers to the same skillet and scrape any browned bits off the bottom. Simmer to reduce the sauce by almost half. Remove from heat and stir in the remaining tablespoon of grapeseed oil.
To serve, divide the cod onto plates, drizzle with the sauce, and sprinkle with parsley.

Notes
Servings: 2-3
Difficulty: Medium
⸎

77. Paleo BLT Frittata

Ingredients
8 eggs
4 slices bacon, cooked and chopped
3-4 cups spinach (or other greens of your choice)
1 large tomato, sliced and seeded
1 tbsp almond milk
1/2 tsp salt
1/4 tsp pepper
2 tbsp chopped fresh basil
1 tbsp extra virgin olive oil

Instructions
Preheat oven to 400 degrees F. In a medium bowl, whisk together the eggs, milk, basil, salt and pepper. Set aside.
Heat olive oil in a 10-inch nonstick skillet over medium heat. Add greens and cook 3-4 minutes until wilted. Add in bacon and stir.
Add egg mixture to the pan and place tomatoes on top. Using a spatula, occasionally lift the edges to allow uncooked egg to run under. When the frittata has set, transfer to the oven and cook for 12-15 minutes or until egg is cooked through. Cut into wedges and serve warm.

Notes
Servings: 5
Difficulty: Easy
⁇

78.   Sausage and Kale "Pasta" Casserole

Ingredients

1 lb. Italian sausage

1 medium spaghetti squash, halved and seeded

Extra virgin olive oil, for drizzling

1 large bunch of kale, de-stemmed, and chopped

1/2 red onion, sliced thin

1/3 cup chicken broth

1/2 cup coconut milk

1 clove garlic, minced

2 tsp Italian seasoning

Salt and freshly ground pepper, to taste

Instructions

Preheat the oven to 400 degrees F. Place the squash in the microwave for 3-4 minutes to soften. Using a sharp knife, cut the squash in half lengthwise. Scoop out the seeds and discard. Place the halves, with the cut side up, on a rimmed baking sheet. Drizzle with olive oil and sprinkle with salt and pepper. Roast in the oven for 45-50 minutes, until you can poke the squash easily with a fork. Let it cool until you can handle it safely. Then scrape the insides with a fork to shred the squash into strands.

Meanwhile, melt the coconut oil in a large oven-safe skillet over medium heat. Add the sausage and brown. Once cooked through, remove to a plate. In the same skillet, add the onion and sauté for 3-4 minutes. Next add the garlic, Italian seasoning, and kale and cook for 2-3 minutes to slightly wilt the kale. Pour in the chicken broth and coconut milk and simmer for an additional 2-3 minutes. Remove from heat. Stir in the cooked sausage. Add the spaghetti squash into the skillet and stir well to combine. Bake for 15-18 minutes, until the top has slightly browned. Serve hot.

Notes

Servings: 4

Difficulty: Medium

⏱

79.   Basic Balsamic Steak Marinade

Ingredients
1 lb. flank steak
Salt and pepper
2 cloves garlic, minced
1/2 tbsp oregano
1/2 tbsp rosemary
1 tsp Paleo mustard
1/4 cup balsamic vinegar
1 tsp honey
1/2 cup extra virgin olive oil

Instructions
Stir together the garlic, oregano, rosemary, mustard, vinegar, honey, and olive oil.
Salt and pepper the steak and place in a shallow dish, then pour the marinade over the steak. Cover and place in the refrigerator for 3-12 hours.
To cook the steak, heat the grill to medium and cook each side approximately 4-5 minutes, or until desired doneness. Let stand for about 5 minutes before slicing and serving.

Notes
Servings: 3
Difficulty: Medium
⁇

80.   Rosemary Beets with Garlicky Kale

Ingredients
6 large leaves of kale (stalks omitted)
3 beets
1 tbsp minced garlic
1 tbsp extra virgin olive oil
1 tsp rosemary (or more, to taste)
Sea salt and pepper, to taste
This recipe makes 3 servings.

Instructions
Preheat oven to 400 degrees Fahrenheit.
Cut stalks and greens off of beets, then peel and chop into 1" cubes.
Mix 1 tbsp olive oil, beet cubes, rosemary, sea salt, and pepper in a large bowl.
Transfer beet mixture to baking dish and bake for 45 minutes, or until beets are tender enough to pierce with a fork.
10 minutes before the beets are ready, rip kale leaves into bite-size pieces.
Add either a small amount of olive oil or water into a pan, and sauté kale and minced garlic on medium heat until wilted.
Place kale onto a plate, and then add the beets on top.
Serve and enjoy!!

Notes
Calories: 123
Total Fat: 5.4g
Saturated Fat: 0.8g
Carbs: 17.9g
Fiber: 3.6g
Protein: 4.1g
⏹

81.   Kale and Red Pepper Frittata

Ingredients
1 tbsp coconut oil
1/2 cup chopped red pepper
1/3 cup chopped onion
3 slices crispy bacon, chopped
2 cups chopped kale, de-stemmed and rinsed
8 large eggs
1/2 cup almond or coconut milk
Salt and pepper to taste

Instructions
Preheat oven to 350 degrees. In a medium bowl, whisk the eggs and milk together. Add salt and pepper. Set aside.
In a non-stick skillet, heat about a tablespoon of coconut oil over medium heat. Add onion and red pepper and sauté for 3 minutes, until onion is translucent. Add kale and cook until it wilts, about 5 minutes.
Add eggs to the pan mixture, along with the bacon. Cook for about 4 minutes until the bottom and edges of the frittata start to set.
Put frittata in the oven and cook for 10-15 minutes until the frittata is cooked all the way through. Slice and serve.

Notes
Servings: 4
Difficulty: Easy
⁇

82. The Best Homemade Ranch Dressing Ever

Ingredients
1/2 cup Paleo mayo (see below)
1/2 cup coconut milk
1/2 tsp onion powder
1 tsp garlic powder
1 tsp dill
Salt and freshly ground pepper, to taste

Instructions
Whisk all ingredients together to combine. Season with salt and pepper to taste. Store in an airtight container in the refrigerator for up to a week.
Mayo recipe
1 egg, room temperature
2 tbsp lemon juice or apple cider vinegar
1/2 tsp salt
1/2 tsp dry mustard
1 cup light olive oil*
In a tall glass (if using an immersion blender) or a blender, place the egg and lemon juice. Let come to room temperature, about one hour. Add the salt and mustard. Blend ingredients.
While blending, very slowly pour in the olive oil. Blend until it reaches desired consistency.
Store in the refrigerator for up to a week.
*It's important to use a light olive oil, not full flavour, for mayonnaise. You could also use almond or walnut oil instead.
⁉

83.   Easy Paleo Slow Cooker Pot Roast

Ingredients
3 lbs. boneless beef roast, trimmed of fat
1 tbsp coconut oil
1 cup beef stock
5 carrots, peeled and diced
2 stalks celery, diced
1/2 large onion, sliced
3 garlic cloves, chopped
1 tbsp fresh parsley, chopped

For the spice rub
1 tbsp freshly ground black pepper
1 tbsp ground coriander
2 tsp cinnamon
1 1/2 tsp salt
1/2 tsp ground clove
1/2 tsp ground allspice

Instructions
Mix together the ingredients for the spice rub and massage into the roast. Heat the coconut oil in a large skillet over medium-high heat. Add the roast to the pan and let sear for 5 minutes. Flip and repeat with the other side. Transfer the roast to the slow cooker.
Add the carrots, onion, garlic, and celery to the slow cooker. Pour in the broth. Turn the heat on to low and cook for 6-7 hours, until the meat is tender. Serve hot sprinkled with chopped parsley.

Notes
Servings: 6
Difficulty: Easy
⁇

84. Spaghetti Squash Shrimp Scampi (Grain-Free & Low Carb)

Ingredients
For the "pasta"
1 spaghetti squash
Extra virgin olive oil, for drizzling
Salt and pepper
1 tsp dried oregano
1 tsp dried basil
For the shrimp scampi
8 oz. shrimp, peeled and deveined
3 tbsp butter
1 tbsp extra virgin olive oil
2 cloves garlic, minced
Pinch of red pepper flakes
Salt and pepper, to taste
1 tbsp fresh parsley, chopped
Juice of 1 lemon
Zest of half a lemon

Instructions
Preheat the oven to 400 degrees F. Place squash in the microwave for 3-4 minutes to soften. Using a sharp knife, cut the squash in half lengthwise. Scoop out the seeds and discard. Place the halves, with the cut side up, on a rimmed baking sheet. Drizzle with olive oil and sprinkle with seasonings. Roast in the oven for 45-50 minutes, until you can poke the squash easily with a fork. Let it cool until you can handle it safely. Then scrape the insides with a fork to shred the squash into strands.
After removing spaghetti squash from the oven, melt the butter and olive oil in a skillet over medium heat. Add in the garlic and sauté for 2-3 minutes. Then add in the shrimp, salt, pepper, and a pinch of red pepper flakes. Cook for 5 minutes, until the shrimp is cooked through. Remove from heat and add in desired amount of cooked spaghetti squash. Toss with lemon juice and zest. Top with parsley to serve.
⯑

85.   Honey Balsamic Roasted Brussels Sprouts

Ingredients
½ lb Brussels sprouts
1 tbsp olive oil
3 tbsp balsamic vinegar
1 tbsp honey
1 tsp garlic powder
1 tsp cayenne pepper
sea salt & black pepper, to taste
This recipe makes 2 servings

Instructions
Preheat oven to 450 degrees Fahrenheit. Line a baking sheet with foil and spray with non-stick cooking spray or spread with a light layer of olive oil.
Halve the Brussels sprouts. Place in a mixing bowl and add in the olive oil, balsamic vinegar, honey, and spices. Toss with hands until fully coated.
Pour Brussels sprouts onto baking sheet in one layer.
Bake for 20 minutes, or until golden brown.
Serve and enjoy! I like to sprinkle another bit of sea salt on them before eating.

Nutrition Facts per serving
Calories: 153
Fat: 7.5g
Saturated Fat: 1.1g
Carbs: 20.5g
Fiber: 4.7g
Protein: 4.2g
⏹

86. Dill & Lemon Baked Salmon in Parchment

Ingredients
2 6-oz. salmon fillets
2 zucchini, halved lengthwise and thinly sliced
1/4 red onion, thinly sliced
1 tsp fresh dill, chopped
2 slices lemon
1 tbsp fresh lemon juice
Extra virgin olive oil, for drizzling
Salt and freshly ground pepper

Instructions
Preheat the oven to 350 degrees F. Prepare two large pieces of parchment paper by folding them in half to crease. Then open the papers and lay flat.
On one side of the crease, place half of the zucchini, red onion, dill, and one lemon slice. Drizzle with olive oil and sprinkle with salt and pepper. Place a salmon fillet on top and drizzle with the lemon juice. Season with salt and pepper. Repeat with the second piece of parchment paper and remaining ingredients.
Fold the parchment paper over the salmon to close, making a half-moon shape. Seal the open sides by folding small pleats in the paper. Place the parchment packets on a rimmed baking sheet and bake for 15-20 minutes until the salmon is opaque. Serve warm.

Notes
Servings: 2
Difficulty: Medium
⁇

DINNER

87.   Balsamic Green Bean Salad

Ingredients
1 1/2 lbs green beans, trimmed and cut to 3 inch long pieces
1/2 red onion, finely chopped
3 tbsp olive oil
2 tbsp balsamic vinegar
1/3 cup chopped walnuts
Salt and pepper to taste

Instructions
Bring a pot of salted water to a boil. Add the green beans and blanch for 2-3 minutes. The beans should be just barely cooked through and still crisp. Prepare a large bowl of ice water while the beans are cooking. Remove beans from hot water and place into ice bath to stop the cooking. Drain.
Place the green beans and red onion in a large bowl. Toss in the olive oil to coat. Sprinkle in the balsamic and season with salt and freshly ground black pepper. Top with chopped walnuts to serve.
☐

88.   Simple Beef and Broccoli Stir Fry

Ingredients
1.5 lbs. sirloin, thinly sliced
4 tbsp coconut aminos, divided
4 tbsp red wine vinegar, divided
3 tbsp chicken broth
4 cloves garlic, minced
1 tsp arrowroot flour
1 tsp honey
1 tbsp ginger, minced
1/2 tsp sesame oil
1 head broccoli, cut into florets
4 carrots, diagonally sliced
3 tbsp coconut oil, divided

Instructions
Place the sirloin in a small bowl with one tablespoon each of red wine vinegar and coconut aminos and toss to coat. Let marinate for 15 minutes at room temperature.

Meanwhile, whisk together 3 tablespoons each red wine vinegar, coconut aminos, and chicken broth. Stir in the garlic, ginger, arrowroot, honey, and sesame oil. Prepare a separate small bowl with 1 tablespoon of water and set it next to the stove along with the garlic sauce.

Melt 2 tablespoons of coconut oil in a large skillet over medium heat. Place the steak in the skillet in a single layer. The meat should sizzle; otherwise the pan is not hot enough. Cook for 1-2 minutes per side to brown, and then transfer to a bowl.

Add the remaining tablespoon of coconut oil to the skillet. Stir in the broccoli and carrots, cooking for 2 minutes. Add the water to the skillet and cover with a lid. Let cook for 2-3 minutes, then remove the lid and cook until all of the water has evaporated.

Add the garlic mixture to the vegetables and stir to coat. Add the beef back into the pan and toss until the sauce thickens and everything is well coated. Serve immediately.

Notes
Servings: 4-6
Difficulty: Medium
?

89.   Homemade Sweet and Salty Paleo Granola

Ingredients
1 cup cashews
3/4 cup almonds
1/4 cup pumpkin seeds, shelled
1/4 cup sunflower seeds, shelled
1/2 cup unsweetened coconut flakes
1/4 cup coconut oil
1/4 cup honey
1 tsp vanilla
1 cup dried cranberries
1 tsp salt

Instructions
Preheat oven to 300 degrees F. Line a baking sheet with parchment paper. Place the cashews, almonds, coconut flakes and pumpkin seeds into a blender and pulse to break the mixture into smaller pieces.
In a large microwave-safe bowl, melt the coconut oil, vanilla, and honey together for 40-50 seconds. Add in the mixture from the blender and the sunflower seeds, and stir to coat.
Spread the mixture out onto the baking sheet and cook for 20-25 minutes, stirring once, until the mixture is lightly browned. Remove from heat. Stir in the dried cranberries and salt.
Press the granola mixture together to form a flat, even surface. Cool for about 15 minutes, and then break into chunks. Store in an airtight container or resealable bag.

Notes
Servings: 6
Difficulty: Easy
⍰

90.   Faux Paleo Napoleon

Ingredients
Dough:
2 ½ cups almond flour
½ teaspoon baking soda
¼ teaspoon sea salt
½ cup + 2 tablespoons organic palm shortening , slightly melted so that it's easy to mix
2 tablespoons honey
1 tablespoon vanilla extract
Filling:
2 cups almond flour
½ cup organic palm shortening or butter (I used shortening. Can't vouch for the results if butter is used, but I don't see why it wouldn't work.)
¼ cup honey
1 tablespoon vanilla extract
⅛ teaspoon sea salt
1 cup chopped fruit of choice for topping

Instruction
Preheat oven to 325 degrees.
Mix all of the dry dough ingredients in a large bowl. Then add in all of the wet dough ingredients. Stir to combine.
Move dough to a silicone baking mat or parchment paper, and roll it out with a rolling pin or something similar. If you need to use your hands, make sure you wet them with water first so that the dough doesn't stick to you.
Using a pastry cutter, cut the dough into 12 equal-sized squares (or rectangles) about 3 (or 2.5) inches wide and 3 inches tall. No need to pull them apart. Once they're done baking, if you can't get them apart easily, just use the pastry cutter again to separate them.
Carefully transfer the baking mat or parchment paper (with the dough on it) to a baking sheet.
Bake for about 10-15 minutes, or until the dough is cooked through and a little bit crispy (like a pie crust would be).
Mix all of the filling ingredients together, except for the fruit.
Once the dough has cooled you can put your layers together. Layer a piece of dough, about 3-4 tablespoons of filling (spread it out), a piece of dough, more filling, a piece of dough, more filling, then some cherries.

Begin a new one. Do this until you run out of dough and filling.

91.   Delish Chicken Soup

Ingredients
5 cups reduced sodium chicken broth
2 cups shredded chicken breast
1 tomato, diced
2 cloves garlic, minced
1-1/2 cups scallions, chopped fine
1/3 cup cilantro, chopped fine
4 lime wedges
2 tsp olive oil
Low sodium salt and fresh pepper to taste
pinch cumin
pinch chilli powder (optional)

Instructions
In a large pot, heat oil over medium heat. Add 1 cup of scallions and garlic. Sauté about 2 minutes then add tomatoes and sauté another minute, until soft.
Add chicken stock, cumin and chilli powder and bring to a boil. Simmer, covered on low for about 15-20 minutes.
Ladle 1 cup chicken broth over the chicken and serve with a lime wedge.
⏺

92.   Chicken Healing Soup

Ingredients
1 teaspoon olive oil
1 cup chopped carrots
1 cup chopped onions
1/2 cup chopped celery
2 cloves garlic, chopped
1-1/2 lbs skinless bone-in chicken breast (makes 14 oz cooked)
7 cups reduced sodium chicken broth
1/4 cup chopped parsley
2 bay leaves
fresh ground black pepper, to taste

Instructions
Heat a large heavy pot on medium heat. Add the oil, carrots, onion, celery and garlic to the pot and stir.
Add chicken, broth, parsley, and bay leaves and bring to a boil. When boiling, reduce heat to low and cover.
Simmer covered over low heat until the chicken and vegetables are tender, about 30 minutes.
Remove the chicken, shred or cut the meat, discard the bones and return the chicken to the pot along with the barley, adjust the low sodium salt if needed and add fresh ground pepper.
Simmer for 20 minutes.... Discard the bay leaves and serve.
⁇

93.   Beautiful Baked Chicken

Ingredients
6 medium bone-in skinless drumsticks
3 tsp low sodium salt
1/2 tsp garlic powder
1/2 tsp paprika
1/2 tsp fresh black pepper
1/2 tsp cayenne pepper
5 tbsp paleo mayonnaise
1 tsp mustard powder
Oil spray
2 teaspoons almond flour

Instructions
Preheat oven to 400°. Line a baking sheet with foil and set a rack above. Spray rack with oil.
Crush cereal in a food processor or chopper. In a bowl mix almond flour with low sodium salt, paprika, garlic powder, black pepper and cayenne pepper. Place in a shallow dish or ziplock bag.
Combine mayonnaise and mustard. Using a cooking brush, brush onto chicken then coat chicken with crushed cereal mixture. Place chicken on wire rack and spray with oil.
Bake 35-40 minutes.
⁈

94.   South American Chicken

Ingredients
1 whole chicken
1/4 cup white vinegar
1 lime, juice of
2 tsp cumin
2 tsp garlic powder
1 tsp dried oregano
Low sodium salt
paprika

Sauce:
2-3 jalapeños, seeded
3 tbsp fresh cilantro
2 tbsp olive oil
1 clove garlic
1 tbsp white vinegar
pinch cumin
low sodium salt and pepper
2 tbsp coconut cream

Instructions
For Sauce:
Place all ingredients in a blender and puree until smooth.
Wash chicken and remove all fat. Place in a large bowl and season generously with beer, vinegar, lime juice, low sodium salt, garlic powder, cumin and oregano. Place in a large bag and marinate overnight. Remove chicken from bag, cut chicken in half and place both halves on a large oven safe baking dish, skin side up. Discard marinade. Sprinkle chicken with paprika and a little more garlic powder and low sodium salt and bake at 425° for about 50 minutes, basting with the pan juices half way through.
⏹

95.   Rosemary Chicken

Ingredients
1 (3 lb) chicken, washed and dried, fat removed
1/2 onion, chopped in large chunks
2 cloves garlic, smashed
1/2 lemon
2-3 sprigs rosemary
1 tbsp herbes de Provence (or dried rosemary)
Low sodium salt and fresh pepper

Instructions
Heat oven to 425°. Season chicken inside and out with low sodium salt, pepper, and herbes de provence. Squeeze lemon juice on the outside of the chicken and stuff the remains of the lemon along with onion, garlic, rosemary sprigs inside the chicken.
Roast the chicken until the internal temperature is 165°F, about 50-60 minutes (Insert thermometer between the leg and the thigh). Let the bird rest for 10 minutes before carving.
Serve with steamed vegetables of choice
⁇

96.   Sexy Sesame Turkey

Ingredients
18 oz turkey breasts
Low sodium salt and pepper to taste
2 tsp sesame oil
2 tsp low sodium soy sauce gluten free
6 tbsp toasted sesame seeds
1/2 tsp low sodium salt
olive oil 2 teaspoons and spray

Instructions
Preheat oven to 425°. Spray a baking sheet with non-stick oil spray.
Combine the sesame oil and soy sauce in a bowl, and the sesame seeds and low sodium salt.
Place turkey in the bowl with the oil and soy sauce, then into the sesame seed mixture to coat well. Place on the baking sheet; lightly spray the top of the chicken with oil spray and bake 8 - 10 minutes. Turn over and cook another 4 - 5 minutes longer or until cooked through.
Serve with cauliflower rice or fried celeriac
⏷

97.   Pollo Al Vinagre

Ingredients
8 lean chicken thighs, skin removed
Low sodium salt and fresh pepper
1/2 cup red wine vinegar
1 cup fat free low salt chicken broth
Stevia to taste
1 tbsp tomato paste
1 tsp butter
1 large shallot, thinly sliced (3/4 cup)
2 cloves garlic, thinly sliced
1/2 cup dry white wine
2 tbsp coconut cream
2 tbsp fresh chopped parsley

Instructions
Season chicken with low sodium salt and pepper.
In a medium saucepan, combine vinegar, stevia, 3/4 cup chicken broth and tomato paste. Boil about 5 minutes, until it reduces down to about 3/4 cup. Remove from heat.
In a large skillet, melt butter over medium-low heat and add chicken. Cook on both sides, until brown, about 6-8 minutes. Remove chicken and set aside. Add the shallots and garlic to the skillet and cook on low until soft, about 5 minutes. Pour the sauce over the chicken, add the wine, remaining broth low sodium salt and pepper. Cover and simmer about 20 minutes until tender.
Remove the chicken, add cream and stir into the sauce (if sauce dries up, add more broth). Boil a few minutes then return chicken to skillet. Top with fresh parsley.
⍰

98.   Chicken Caully Delish

Ingredients
1 1/2 tbsp olive oil
2 large chicken breast halves, bone in, skin removed
Low sodium salt and pepper to taste
1/2 medium head of cauliflower, cut into florets (about 4 cups)
1 medium onion, sliced thinly
4 cloves of garlic, sliced thinly
1driedchilli pepper, sliced
1/3 cup dry white wine
1 cup reduced sodium chicken stock
1 sprig rosemary, needles removed and roughly chopped, plus additional for garnish

Instructions
Pre-heat oven to 375°F. Cut chicken in half to make 4 pieces, leaving the bone on.
Heat oil in a large, oven safe sauté pan with straight sides over medium-high heat. Season the chicken with low sodium salt and pepper and brown 2-3 minutes per side. Remove chicken and set aside.
Lower heat to medium and add onion, cauliflower florets, garlic and chill …Sauté, stirring frequently, for 2-3 minutes until vegetables start to brown.
Add the white wine, cherry peppers and additional optional liquid. Raise heat and allow to boil for about 2 minutes before adding chicken stock. Add chicken breasts back into pan, bone side down, sprinkle rosemary on top, bring to a boil and then place the pan in the oven, uncovered.
Cook for 20-25 minutes or until chicken reaches 165°F.
Remove from oven carefully, with towel or kitchen gloves, serve and enjoy!
⁇

99.   Courgette Spaghetti with Delish Chicken

Ingredients

2 skinless chicken breast halves, diced in 1 inch cubes

cooking spray

1/2 tsp each of dried oregano and dries basil

Low sodium salt and fresh pepper

2 courgettes spiralized

2 cups grape tomatoes, halved

6 cloves garlic, smashed and coarsely chopped

4 tsp extra virgin olive oil

4 tbsp chopped fresh basil

Instructions

Bring a large pot of salted water to boil.

Season chicken generously with low sodium salt, pepper, oregano and basil. Heat a large skillet on high heat. When hot, spray with oil and add chicken. Cook about 3-4 minutes, until no longer pink. Remove chicken and set aside.

Add courgette pasta and cook according to package directions. Reserve about 1/2 cup pasta water before draining.

While pasta cooks, add olive oil to skillet on high heat. Add garlic and sauté until golden brown (do not burn).

Add tomatoes, low sodium salt and pepper and reduce heat to medium-low. Sauté about 4-5 minutes. When pasta is drained, add pasta to tomatoes and toss well. If pasta seems too dry, add some of the reserved pasta water.

Add fresh basil and chicken and toss well. Serve and top with dried garlic powder and the rest of the basil.
⁂

100. Chicken Pea Stir Fry

Ingredients
For the sauce:
1 tbsp low sodium soy sauce gluten free
1 tbsp fresh lime juice
2 tbsp water

For the Stir Fry:
1 lb skinless, boneless chicken breast, sliced thin
Low sodium salt, to taste
1 tbsp sesame oil,
2 tsp fresh garlic, minced
1 tsp fresh ginger, grated
2 cups sugar snap peas
1 cup carrots, sliced diagonally
scallions for garnish

Instructions
Combine soy sauce, lime juice, water in a small bowl, mix together and set aside.
Season chicken lightly with low sodium salt. Heat a large wok over high heat. When the wok is very hot, add half of the oil, then add the chicken. Stir fry, stirring occasionally until the chicken is cooked through and browned, about 3-4 minutes. With a slotted spoon, remove the chicken and set aside. Reduce heat to medium.
Add the remaining oil to the wok; add the garlic and ginger, stir for 20 seconds. Add the sugar snap peas and carrots, stirring over medium high heat until tender crisp, about 3-4 minutes.
Return the chicken to the wok, add the soy sauce-lime mixture, mix well and cook another 30 seconds to one minute. Serve immediately and top with fresh scallions.
⁇

101. Scrumptious Cod in Delish Sauce

Ingredients
1 lb. cod fillets
1/3 cup almond flour
1/2 tsp low sodium salt
2-3 tbsp extra virgin olive oil
2 tbsp walnut oil, divided
3/4 cup low sodium chicken stock
3 tbsp lemon juice
1/4 cup capers, drained
2 tbsp fresh parsley, chopped

Instructions
Stir the almond flour and low sodium salt together in a shallow bowl. Rinse off the fish and pat dry with a paper towel. Dredge the fish in the almond flour mixture to coat.
Heat enough olive oil to coat the bottom of a large skillet over medium-high heat along with one tablespoon walnut oil. Working in batches, add the cod and cook for 2-3 minutes per side to brown. Remove to a plate and set aside.
Add the chicken stock, lemon juice, and capers to the same skillet and scrape any browned bits off the bottom. Simmer to reduce the sauce by almost half. Remove from heat and stir in the remaining tablespoon of walnut oil.
To serve, divide the cod onto plates, drizzle with the sauce, and sprinkle with parsley.
▢

102. Delish Baked dill Salmon

Ingredients
2 6-oz. salmon fillets
2 zucchini, halved lengthwise and thinly sliced
1/4 red onion, thinly sliced
1 tsp fresh dill, chopped
2 slices lemon
1 tbsp fresh lemon juice
Extra virgin olive oil, for drizzling
low sodium salt and freshly
ground pepper

Instructions
Preheat the oven to 350 degrees F. Prepare a baking tray
Place half of the zucchini, red onion, dill, and one lemon slice. Drizzle with olive oil and sprinkle with low sodium salt and pepper. Place a salmon fillet on top and drizzle with the lemon juice. Season with low sodium salt and pepper. Repeat with the remaining ingredients.
Bake for 15-20 minutes until the salmon is opaque.
⏺

103. Prawn garlic Fried "Rice"

Ingredients
1 tbsp coconut oil
1 cup white onion, finely chopped
2 cloves garlic, minced
8 oz. prawns peeled and deveined
1 medium carrot, chopped
1/2 cup peas
2 cups cooked cauliflower rice
2 eggs, beaten
Low sodium salt and pepper, to taste

Instructions
Heat a wok or large pan over medium-high heat. Melt the coconut oil and add the onion and garlic to the pan.
Cook for 3-4 minutes until the onion starts to soften. Add the shrimp and cook for 1 minute.
Add the carrot, peas, and bell pepper to the pan. Cook for 3-4 minutes, and then stir in the cauliflower rice.
Clear a circle in the center of the pan and pour in the beaten eggs. Stir to scramble the eggs and then combine with the other ingredients.
Season with low sodium salt and pepper to taste
⬚

104. Tasty Tomato Tilapia

Ingredients
2 tbsp extra virgin olive oil
4 (6 oz) tilapia filets
2 garlic cloves, crushed
2 shallots, minced
2 tomatoes, chopped
2 tbsp capers
1/4 cup white wine
Low sodium salt and fresh pepper

Instructions
Brush fish with 1 tbsp olive and season with low sodium salt and pepper.
In a medium sauté pan, heat remaining olive oil. Add garlic and shallots and sauté on medium-low about 4-5 minutes. Add tomatoes and season with low sodium salt and pepper. Add wine and sauté until wine reduces, about 5 minutes. Add capers and sauté an additional minute.
Meanwhile, set broiler to low and place fish about 8 inches from the flame. Broil until fish is cooked through, about 7 minutes.
Place fish on a platter and top with tomato caper sauce.
Eat with a green salad and paleo dressing
⏺

105. Prawn Asparagus Stir Fry

Ingredients

2 tbsp low sodium soy sauce (use tamari for gluten free)

1 tsp sherry

1 tbsp grated peeled fresh ginger

2 tsp sesame oil

1 pound asparagus, trimmed and cut diagonally into 2-inch pieces

1 chili pepper, sliced

2 cloves garlic, chopped

1 bell pepper, sliced

1 lb large tiger prawns, cleaned

Low sodium salt and pepper to taste

Instructions

Stir together soy sauce, sherry and ginger; set aside.

In a wok, heat 1 tsp sesame oil over medium-high heat until hot. Add prawns and cook until white, about 3 minutes. Remove from wok and set aside.

Add remaining oil to wok. When oil is hot, add asparagus and cook 5 minutes or until tender-crisp, stirring frequently. Add garlic. Add peppers and stir another minute.

Add prawns back into the wok. Pour sauce over everything and mix another minute. Adjust low sodium salt and pepper to taste.

Serve with cauliflower rice

[?]

106. Cilantro Fish Delish

Ingredients
1 1/2 pounds fresh cod or any white fish
1/4 teaspoon plus 1/8 teaspoon ground cumin
Low sodium salt and freshly ground black pepper
2 teaspoons extra-virgin olive oil
5 garlic cloves, crushed
2 tablespoons lime juice (from 1 medium lime)
3 to 4 tablespoons chopped fresh cilantro

Instructions
Season the fish with cumin, and low sodium salt and pepper to taste.
Heat a large nonstick skillet over medium-high heat. Add 1 teaspoon of the oil to the pan, then add half of the fish. Cook them undisturbed for about 2 minutes. Turn the shrimp over and cook until opaque throughout, about 1 minute. Transfer to a plate.
Add the remaining 1 teaspoon oil and the remaining fish to the pan and cook, undisturbed, for about 2 minutes.
Turn the shrimp over, add the garlic, and cook until the shrimp is opaque throughout, about 1 minute.
Return the first batch to the skillet, mix well so that the garlic is evenly incorporated and remove the pan from the heat.
Squeeze the lime juice over all the shrimp. Add the cilantro, toss well, and serve with cauliflower rice
⁉

107. Perfect Prawns

Ingredients
2 tsp extra virgin olive oil
1.25 lb large or jumbo prawns, peeled and deveined (1 lb after peeled)
6 garlic cloves, chopped
1 tsp crushed red pepper flakes
fresh pepper to taste
2 tablespoons of capers (rinsed)
1/4 cup of white wine
1 cup clam juice
juice from one lemon
generous handful of chopped parsley
celeriac mash see below

Instructions
Heat olive oil in a skillet. Add garlic, pepper flakes, and sauté 2-3 minutes.
Add wine, clam juice, lemon juice, parsley, low sodium salt and pepper, and stir. Cook for another 2-3 minutes.
Add prawns and cook for 2-3 minutes. Do not overcook or it will become tough and chewy. Serve with liquid in a bowl and some celeriac mash (boil 3 cups diced celeriac for 10 minutes and blend with olive oil and garlic powder)
⍰

108. Fish Fillet Delux

Ingredients
4 white fish fillets, about 5 oz each
4 tsp olive oil
Low sodium salt and fresh pepper, to taste
4 sprigs fresh herbs (parsley, rosemary, oregano)
1 lemon, sliced thin
4 large pieces heavy duty aluminum foil,

Instructions
Place the fish in the center of the foil, season with low sodium salt and pepper and drizzle with olive oil. Place a slice of lemon on top of each piece of fish, then a sprig of herbs on each. Fold up the edges so that it's completely sealed and no steam will escape, creating a loose tent.
Heat half of the grill (on one side) on high heat with the cover closed. When the grill is hot, place the foil packets on the side of the grill with the burners off (indirect heat) and close the grill. Depending on the thickness of your fish, cook 10 to 15 minutes, or until the fish is opaque and cooked through.....serve with green salad and paleo dressing.
⁇

109. Gambas Ajillo

Ingredients
1 lb large shrimp, peeled and deveined (weight after you peel them)
6 cloves garlic, sliced thin
1 tbsp Spanish olive oil
crushed red pepper flakes
pinch paprika
low sodium salt

Instructions
In a large skillet, heat oil on medium heat and add the garlic and red pepper flakes. Sauté until golden, about 2 minutes being careful not to burn.
 Add shrimp and season with salt and paprika. Cook 2-3 minutes until shrimp is cooked through. Do not overcook or it will become tough and chewy.
See previous recipe for celeriac mash!
⬚

110.   Tantalizing Tuna Steak

Ingredients
16 oz sushi grade tuna
1 tsp toasted sesame oil
Low sodium salt
fresh pepper
4 cups arugula

For the soy-ginger vinaigrette:
1 tbsp minced ginger
1 tbsp minced green onion
1 tbsp minced garlic
1/2 cup balsamic vinegar
1/4 cup red wine
1/4 cup soy sauce low sodium gluten free
Stevia to taste
2 tsp toasted sesame oil
1 tsp mustard powder

Instructions
Rub the tuna steaks with 1 tsp oil, and sprinkle with low sodium salt and pepper. Place the tuna steaks in a very hot saute pan and cook for only 1 minute on each side. Set aside on a platter.
Meanwhile, prepare salad and soy vinaigrette. Lightly coat salad with vinaigrette. Slice tuna steaks and place on top of arugula. Drizzle additional vinaigrette over the top.
⁇

111. Avocado Salad with Cilantro and Lime

Ingredients
Turkey Breast chopped
Two avocados, diced
2/3 green cabbage, chopped
5 green onions (scallions), white and pale green parts, minced
Juice of 2 limes
Two handfuls of fresh cilantro, chopped
low sodium salt to taste
One large English Cucumber

Instructions
Mix all ingredients except cucumber -slice it thinly and use it as a base for the salad. For "party style",
slice 1-2 inch sections, scoop out the center with a grapefruit spoon, and fill the cucumber "cups" with the
salad.
Divine Dressing:
Mix together, 4 Tbsp. chili powder, 1 tsp each garlic powder, onion powder, and oregano, 2 tsp each
paprika and cumin, 4 tsp low sodium salt, and 1/8-1/4 tsp red pepper flakes.
Add 1 cup olive oil and half cup rice vinegar.
⁂

112.   Mexican Medley Salad

Ingredients
For the Chicken or turkey:
1 lb boneless chicken/turkey breasts
1 tbsp olive oil
low sodium salt and pepper, to taste

For the Salsa:
1 large tomato, quartered
1/2 red onion, cut into large chunks
1 jalapeno pepper, stem and seeds removed and halved
1 garlic clove, peeled
1 small bunch of cilantro leaves
Juice of 1 lime
low sodium salt and pepper, to taste

Instructions
Preheat oven to 375 F.
Brush chicken breasts on both sides with olive oil and sprinkle with low sodium salt and pepper. Bake on a baking sheet for 35 to 40 minutes, until no longer pink in the center.
While chicken is baking, add all salsa ingredients to a food processor and pulse using the chopping blade until finely chopped.
Transfer the salsa to a large bowl and clean out the food processor. You will be using it to shred the chicken.
Remove chicken from the oven and allow to cool. Once cool enough to handle, cut each breast into three or four smaller pieces and add to the food processor. Pulse using the chopping blade until shredded.
Add chicken to bowl with salsa and mix well with a fork.
Refrigerate for at least two hours until chicken salad is chilled.
⍰

113. Artichoke Heart & Turkey Salad Radicchio Cups

Ingredients

1.5 cups diced cooked turkey

¼ cup finely diced red onion

1 small carrot julienned and cut into small pieces (or ½ a diced red bell pepper)

4-5 artichoke hearts (I used canned in water) diced low sodium salt and pepper to taste.

6 Radicchio leaves

Instructions

Place all ingredients, except the radicchio leaves in a large bowl and combine.

Place a scoop if salad into each Radicchio cup and serve.

Store salad in an air tight container in the fridge.

Divine Dressing:

Mix together, 4 Tbsp. chili powder, 1 tsp each garlic powder, onion powder, and oregano, 2 tsp each paprika and cumin, 4 tsp low sodium salt, and 1/8-1/4 tsp red pepper flakes. Add 1 cup olive oil and half cup rice vinegar.

⏴

114. Tempting Tuna Stuffed Tomato

Ingredients
2 large tomatoes
Lettuce leaves (optional)
2 (5 or 6 oz.) cans wild albacore tuna
1 stalk celery, chopped
1/2 small onion, chopped
1/4 tsp. low sodium salt
1/4 tsp. ground black pepper

Instructions
Wash and dry the tomatoes and remove any stem.
Arrange the tomatoes on a plate on top of lettuce leaves (optional).
Combine the remaining ingredients in a mixing bowl and add additional low sodium salt and/or pepper if desired.
Spoon into the tomatoes and serve.
⁇

115. Incredibly Delish Avocado Tuna Salad

Ingredients
1 avocado
1 lemon, juiced, to taste
1 tablespoon chopped onion, to taste
5 ounces cooked or canned wild tuna
low sodium salt and pepper to taste

Instructions
Cut the avocado in half and scoop the middle of both avocado halves into a bowl, leaving a shell of avocado flesh about 1/4-inch thick on each half.
Add lemon juice and onion to the avocado in the bowl and mash together.
Add tuna, low sodium salt and pepper, and stir to combine. Taste and adjust if needed.
Fill avocado shells with tuna salad and serve.
⬚

116. Italian Tuna Bonanza Salad

Ingredients
10 sun-dried tomatoes
2 (5 oz) can of tuna
1-2 ribs of celery, diced finely
2 Tablespoons of extra virgin olive oil
1 cloves garlic, minced
3 Tablespoons finely chopped parsley
1/2 Tablespoon lemon juice
low sodium salt and pepper to taste

Instructions
Prepare the sun-dried tomatoes by softening them in warm water for 30 minutes until soft. Then, pat the tomatoes dry and chop finely.
Flake the tuna. and mix the tuna together with the chopped tomatoes, celery, extra virgin olive oil, garlic, parsley, and lemon juice. Add low sodium salt and pepper to taste.
If not serving immediately, mix with extra olive oil just before serving.
Optional: Make cucumber boats with them.
⧉

117. Tasty Carrot Salad

Ingredients
5 carrots, medium
1 tbs. whole black mustard seeds
1/4 tsp. low sodium salt
2 tsp. lemon juice
2 tbs. olive oil
Add 1 Grated egg on top

Instructions
Trim and peel and grate carrots. In a bowl, toss with low sodium salt and set aside.
In a small heavy pan over medium heat, heat oil.
When very hot, add mustard seeds. As soon as the seeds begin to pop, in a few seconds, pour oil and seeds over carrots.
Add lemon juice and toss. Serve at room temperature or cold.

Add Grated egg.

⬚

118. Creamy Carrot Salad
Ingredients
1 pound carrots - shredded
20 ounces crushed pineapple -- drained
8 ounces Coconut milk
3/4 cup flaked coconut
Stevia to taste
Shredded turkey one breast
Instructions
Combine all ingredients, tossing well. Cover and chill.

⬚

119. Sea Scallops Sensation
Ingredients
For the dressing:
1 tbsp red wine vinegar
1 tbsp cider vinegar
2 tbsp olive oil
1 tsp minced shallots
4 drops tbsp stevia
For the salad:
2 cups diced cooked and peeled beets
12 large sea scallops (18 oz)
olive oil cooking spray
low sodium salt and pepper to taste
5 oz baby arugula
8 grape tomatoes, halved
Instructions
Cover the beets with water in a medium pot and bring to a boil. Cover and cook over medium-low heat until tender when pierced with a fork, about 50 to 60 minutes. Peel and dice into small cubes; set aside to cool.

Season scallops with low sodium salt and pepper. Heat a large nonstick pan on a medium-high heat. When the pan is hot, spray with oil and place scallops in the pan. Sear without touching them until the bottom forms a nice caramel coloured crust, about 2 to 3 minutes. Turn and cook until their centers are still slightly translucent (you can check this by viewing them from the side), about 1 to 2 more minutes, careful not to overcook. Remove from the pan.

Make vinaigrette by whisking the dressing ingredients in a small bowl. Toss with the arugula. Evenly divide the arugula between four large plates. Top each with 1/2 cup beet, tomato and 3 scallops each. Serve immediately.

⁇

120. Pure Delish Spinach Salad

Ingredients
2 bunches fresh spinach
1 bunch scallions, chopped
juice of 1 lemon
1/4 tbsp olive oil
pepper to taste
optional: rice vinegar to taste

Instructions
Wash spinach well. Drain and chop.
After a few minutes, squeeze excess water.
Add scallions, lemon juice, oil and pepper.
⏴

121. Mouthwatering Mushroom Salad

Ingredients
2/3 cup olive oil
1/3 cup fresh lemon juice
One tablespoon red wine vinegar
1 tsp dried thyme
pepper and garlic powder to taste
1 pound fresh mushrooms, thinly sliced
1/4 cup minced parsley
Rucola leaves

Instructions
Combine all ingredients except the mushrooms, parsley and greens, and mix well.
Add the mushrooms and toss with 2 forks. Cover and let stand at room temperature.
At serving time, drain and sprinkle with the parsley. Pile in a serving dish lined with greens.
⏴

122. Skinny Sweet Potato Salad

Ingredients
4 small sweet potatoes
1 tablespoon olive oil extra virgin
1 teaspoon mustard powder
4 celery stalks, sliced 1/4-inch thick
1 small red bell pepper, cut into 1/4-inch dice
2 scallions, finely chopped
low sodium salt and pepper
1/2 cup coarsely chopped toasted pecans
Chopped fresh chives

Instructions
Preheat oven to 400°F.
Wrap each sweet potato in foil and bake for 1 hour.
Unwrap; let cool. Peel; cut into 3/4-inch chunks.
In a large bowl, mix oil and mustard. Add sweet potatoes, celery,
red pepper and scallions; toss gently.
Season to taste with low sodium salt and pepper.
Cover and refrigerate about 1 hour.
Fold in pecans and sprinkle with chives.
？

123. Roasted Lemon Herb Chicken

Ingredients
12 total pieces bone-in chicken thighs and legs
1 medium onion, thinly sliced
1 tbsp dried rosemary
1 tsp dried thyme
1 lemon, sliced thin
1 orange, sliced thin
For the marinade:
5 tbsp extra virgin olive oil
6 cloves garlic, minced
Stevia to taste
Juice of 1 lemon
Juice of 1 orange
1 tbsp Italian seasoning
1 tsp onion powder
Dash of red pepper flakes
low sodium salt and freshly ground pepper, to taste

Instructions
Whisk together all of the marinade ingredients in a small bowl. Place the chicken in a baking dish (or a large Ziploc bag) and pour the marinade over it. Marinate for 3 hours to overnight.
Preheat the oven to 400 degrees F. Place the chicken in a baking dish and arrange with the onion, orange, and lemon slices.
Sprinkle with thyme, rosemary, low sodium salt and pepper. Cover with aluminum foil and bake for 30 minutes.
Remove the foil, baste the chicken, and bake for another 30 minutes uncovered, until the chicken is cooked through.
⁇

124. Basil Turkey with Roasted Tomatoes

Ingredients
2 turkey breasts
1 cup mushrooms, chopped
1/2 medium onion, chopped
1-2 tbsp extra virgin olive oil
Half cup thinly sliced fresh basil
low sodium salt and pepper, to taste
1 pint cherry tomatoes
Stevia to taste
Fresh parsley, for garnish

Instructions
Preheat the oven to 400 degrees F. Place the tomatoes on a baking sheet and drizzle with olive oil and stevia. Sprinkle with low sodium salt and pepper and toss to coat evenly. Bake for 15-20 minutes until soft. While the tomatoes are roasting, heat one tablespoon of olive oil in a large pan over low heat. Add the onions and mushrooms and cook for 10-12 minutes to soften and caramelize, stirring regularly. Clear a space for the chicken.
Season the turkey with low sodium salt and pepper and then place it in the pan. Simmer for 15 minutes or until the chicken is cooked through. Every 5 minutes or so, spoon the sauce in the pan over the turkey.
To assemble, divide the tomatoes between two plates. Place one turkey breast on each and then spoon the onions, mushrooms, and pan drippings over the turkey. Garnish with parsley.
⁇

125. Cheeky Chicken Salad

Ingredients
olive oil spray
2 tsp olive oil
16 oz (2 large) skinless boneless chicken breasts, cut into 24 1-inch chunks
Low sodium salt and pepper to taste
4 cups shredded romaine
1 cup shredded red cabbage

For the Skinny Cheeky Sauce
2 1/2 tbsppaleo mayonnaise
2 tbsp scallions, chopped fine plus more for topping
1 1/2 tspchilli flakes

Instructions
Preheat oven to 425°F. Spray a baking sheet with olive oil spray.
Season chicken with low sodium salt and pepper, olive oil and mix well so the olive oil evenly coats all of the chicken.
Meanwhile combine the sauce in a medium bowl. When the chicken is ready, drizzle it over the top and enjoy!!
⁇

126. Melting Mustard Chicken

Ingredients
8 small chicken thighs, skin removed
3 tsp mustard powder
1 tbsppaleo mayonnaise
1 clove garlic, crushed
1 lime, squeezed, and lime zest
3/4 tsp pepper
Low sodium salt
dried parsley

Instructions
Preheat oven to 400°. Rinse the chicken and remove the skin and all fat. Pat dry ...place in a large bowl and season generously with low sodium salt.
In a small bowl combine mustard, mayonnaise, lime juice, lime zest, garlic and pepper. Mix well.
Pour over chicken, tossing well to coat.
Spray a large baking pan with a little Pam to prevent sticking since all the fat and skin was removed from chicken. Place chicken to fit in a single layer.
Top the chicken with dried parsley. Bake until cooked through, about 30-35 minutes.
Finish the chicken under the broiler until it is golden brown. Serve chicken with the pan juices drizzled over the top.
🔲

127. Tantalizing Turkey with Roasted Vegetables

Ingredients
10 (20 oz) Turkey Breasts
20 medium asparagus, ends trimmed, cut in half
3 red bell peppers
1 cup carrots, sliced in half long way
2 red onions, chopped in large chunks
10 oz sliced mushrooms
1/2 cup plus 2 tbsp rice vinegar
1/4 cup extra virgin olive oil
1 tsp stevia
Low sodium salt and pepper
3 tbsp fresh rosemary
2 cloves garlic, smashed and sliced
2 tbsp oregano or thyme
4 leaves fresh sage, chopped

Instructions
Preheat oven to 425°. Wash and dry the chicken well with a paper towel. Combine all the ingredients together and using your hands and arrange in a very large roasting pan.
The vegetables should not touch the turkey or it will steam instead of roast.
All ingredients should be spread out in a single layer. If necessary, use two baking sheets or disposable tins to achieve this. Bake for 35 - 40 minutes.
⁊

128. Chicken a la King

Ingredients
6 chicken thighs, skin and fat removed
olive oil spray
1 red bell pepper, chopped
1 cup chopped mushrooms
1/2 onion, chopped
2 garlic cloves, finely chopped
1 (28-ounce) can crushed tomatoes
1/4 cup fat free chicken broth, more if needed
1 tsp dried oregano leaves
1/4 cup fresh chopped basil leaves
Low sodium salt and freshly ground black pepper

Instructions
Season chicken with low sodium salt and pepper. In a large heavy saute pan, heat the pan over a medium-high flame and spray with cooking oil.
Add the chicken pieces to the pan and saute just until brown, about 3-4 minutes per side.
Add the peppers, onion and garlic to the pan and saute over medium heat until the onion is tender, about 3-4 minutes, then add mushrooms and cook another 2-3 minutes. Season with low sodium salt and pepper. Add the tomatoes, broth, and oregano.
Cover the pan and bring the sauce to a simmer. Continue simmering over low heat until the chicken is just cooked through, about 25 minutes.
Add the chopped basil 5 minutes before sauce is done.
Option – serve with cauliflower rice!
⁇

129. Chicken Peanut Lettuce Wraps

Ingredients
For the Peanut Sauce:
1/2 cup reduced-sodium chicken broth
3 tbsp PB2 (or 2 tbsp peanut butter)
Stevia to taste
1 tbsp soy sauce (use Tamari for gluten free)
1/2 tbsp freshly grated ginger
1 clove garlic, crushed
For the Chicken cooking spray
16 oz ground chicken
4 cloves garlic, crushed
1 tbsp fresh ginger, grated
1 tbsp soy sauce (use Tamari for gluten free)
3/4 cups shredded carrots
2/3 cup scallions, chopped
3/4 cup shredded red cabbage
2 tbsp chopped peanuts
cilantro leaves, for garnish
4 lime wedges
8 iceberg lettuces outer leaves

Instructions
Make the peanut sauce; in a small saucepan combine chicken broth, stevia, 1 tablespoon soy sauce, 1/2 tablespoon fresh ginger, and 1 clove crushed garlic and simmer over medium-low heat stirring occasionally until sauce becomes smooth and thickens, about 6 to 8 minutes.
Meanwhile, heat a large non-stick skillet or wok over high medium until hot. When hot, spray with oil and sauté the chicken until cooked through and browned, breaking it up as it cooks; add the remaining garlic and ginger and saute 1 minute. Add the tablespoon of soy sauce, cook 1 minute.
Add the shredded carrots, and 1/2 cup of the scallions and sauté until tender crisp, about 1-2 minutes. Set aside.
Divide the chicken equally between 8 lettuce leaves, top each with shredded cabbage, remaining scallions, drizzle with peanut sauce, chopped peanuts and cilantro, for garnish and serve with lime wedges.

130. Highly Delish Herb Salmon

Ingredients
4 garlic cloves
1 tsp dried Herbs de Provence
1 tsp red wine vinegar
1 tsp olive oil
2 tbsp mustard powder
olive oil spray
4 (6 oz) wild salmon fillets, 1" thick (if frozen, thaw first)
Low sodium salt and fresh ground pepper to taste
4 lemon wedges for serving

Instructions
In a mini food processor, or using a mortar and pestle mash garlic with the herbs, vinegar, oil, and mustard until it becomes a paste. Set aside.
Season salmon with a pinch of low sodium salt and fresh pepper. Heat a grill or grill pan over high heat until hot. Spray the pan lightly with oil and reduce the heat to medium-low. Place the salmon on the hot grill pan and cook without moving for 5 minutes.
Turn and cook the other side for an additional 3-4 minutes spooning on half of the garlic herb mustard sauce.
Turn and cook 1 more-minute spooning the other side of the fish with remaining sauce. Turn once again and let the fish finish cooking about one more minute.
Serve with a green salad and paleo dressing
⁇

131. Happy Halibut Soup

Ingredients
1 tsp olive oil
2 chopped shallots
2 cloves of garlic
3 medium diced tomatoes
4 oz cup of white wine
1 cup clam juice
2 cups vegetable stock
3/4 lb halibut filet, skin removed cut into large pieces
1 dozen small clams
pinch of saffron
1/4 cup fresh chopped parsley

Instructions
Add olive oil to a large heavy pot; over medium heat sautée shallots and garlic until translucent. Add the tomatoes, wine, clam juice and the bone from the halibut if you have one. Add vegetable stock, saffron, fresh thyme and stir.
Add the clams; cover and cook 2 minutes, add the fish and cook and additional 3 minutes, or until the shrimp turns pink and the clams open.
⁇

132. Tasty Teriyaki Salmon

Ingredients

3 tbsp low-sodium soy sauce (or tamari for gluten free)

3 tbsp mirin (Japanese sweet rice wine)

3 tbsp sake

Stevia to taste

1 lb fresh wild salmon fillet, cut in 4 pieces

2 tsp cooking oil

Instructions

Combine the soy sauce, mirin, sake, and stevia in a resealable bag. Add the salmon and mix to coat. Refrigerate for 1 hour or up to 8 hours.

Remove salmon, reserving the marinade. Heat a frying pan or sauté pan over medium-high heat. When hot, swirl in the oil.

Sear salmon, 2 minutes per side. Turn heat to low and pour in the reserved marinade. Cover and cook for 4 to 5 minutes, until cooked through.

Serve with cauliflower rice

⁇

133. Sexy Shrimp Cakes

Ingredients
1 lb shrimp, peeled and deveined (weight after peeled)
1 large jalapeño, seeded and minced (for spicy, leave the seeds)
1 garlic clove, minced
3 medium scallions, chopped
2 tablespoons fresh cilantro, chopped
1/4 teaspoon low sodium salt
1/8 teaspoon fresh ground black pepper
1 tablespoon almond flour for binding

For topping:
4 lime wedges
1/2 medium avocado, sliced thin

Instructions
Dry shrimp well with a paper towel then place the shrimp in the food processor along with jalapeño and garlic then pulse a few times until almost pasty.
Combine the shrimp in a large bowl with remaining ingredients and mix well to combine.
Using rubber gloves (easier with gloves), form shrimp into 4 patties.
Heat a non-stick skillet over medium heat and spray with oil. Add the shrimp cakes to the heated grill and cook 4 minutes without disturbing, then gently flip and cook an additional 4 minutes.
Serve with fresh lime juice and celeriac mash – see recipe above
🔲

134. SEXY SEARED Scampi

Ingredients
2 tsp olive oil
1 1/2 lbs shrimp, peeled and deveined (weight after peeled)
1/4 tsp low sodium salt
1/4 tsp ground black pepper
1/4 tsp crushed red pepper
2 tbsp dry parsley
lemon wedges

Instructions
Heat 1 tsp oil in 12 inch skillet over high heat until smoking. Meanwhile, toss shrimp with low sodium salt and pepper.
Add half of the shrimp to the pan in single layer and cook until edges turn pink, about 1 minute.
Remove pan from heat, flip shrimp using tongs and let it stand about 30 seconds until all of the shrimp is opaque except for the center.
Transfer to a plate and repeat with the second batch and the remaining teaspoon of oil. After second batch has stood off the heat, add the first batch to the pan and toss to combine.
Cover skillet and let shrimp stand for 1 - 2 minutes. Shrimp will now be cooked through. Serve immediately with a green salad and lemon wedges
☐

135. Skinny Chicken salad

Ingredients
Salad:
1 small head (or 4 cups) savoy cabbage, finely shredded –
1 cup carrot, julienned
1/4 cup scallions, trimmed and julienned
1/4 cup radishes, julienned
1/4 cup fresh cilantro, chopped
1/4 cup fresh mint, chopped
2 cups cooked organic chicken

Vinaigrette:
2 tablespoons coconut or rice vinegar
2 tablespoons sesame oil (use unrefined, expeller or cold-pressed)
juice of 1/2 a lime
1 chipotle pepper
1 clove garlic, crushed
1 teaspoon fresh ginger, grated

Instructions
Salad – Combine cabbage, carrots, scallions and radishes. Top with chicken, cilantro and mint and set aside.
Vinaigrette –Combine the vinaigrette ingredients. Taste to see if it needs any adjustments. If it is too spicy, you can add more lime juice to counteract it.
Drizzle salad with vinaigrette & enjoy.
⏀

136. Spectacular Spinach Omelet

Ingredients
2 eggs
1.5 cups raw spinach
coconut oil, about 1 tbsp
1/3 c tomatoes and onion salsa (lightly fried in pan)
1 tbsp fresh cilantro

Instructions
Melt coconut oil on medium in frying pan. Add spinach, cook until mostly wilted. Beat eggs and add to pan.
Flip once the egg sets around the edge. When it's almost done add the salsa on top just to warm it. Move to plate and add cilantro. Serves one.
⏎

137. Blushing Blueberry Omelet

Ingredients
2 eggs
1 tsp. vanilla extract
coconut oil
1/2 c. blueberries
Stevia to taste

Instructions
Lightly beat two eggs and vanilla extract in a bowl. Heat 6" non-stick pan over medium heat.
While pan is heating, heat half the blueberries in a saucepan until juices flow.
Add coconut oil to non-stick pan and coat evenly.
When thoroughly heated, add egg mixture. Swish once and let sit.
When eggs are about 70% settled, swish again. There should be a nice crispy layer around the side of the pan.
When it starts to separate from the side, add fresh and cooked blueberries to omelet, reserving a few for garnish.
Crispy layer should really be pulling away from pan now.
 Use a fork to help fold the omelet over. Slide on to plate, top with reserved blueberry filling, and enjoy
⏺

138. Paleo Shrimp Fried "Rice"

Ingredients
1 tbsp coconut oil
1 cup white onion, finely chopped
2 cloves garlic, minced
8 oz. shrimp, peeled and deveined
1 medium carrot, chopped
1/2 cup peas
1/4 cup red bell pepper, finely chopped
2 cups cooked cauliflower rice
2 eggs, beaten
Salt and pepper, to taste

Instructions
Heat a wok or large pan over medium-high heat. Melt the coconut oil and add the onion and garlic to the pan. Cook for 3-4 minutes until the onion starts to soften. Add the shrimp and cook for 1 minute.
Add the carrot, peas, and bell pepper to the pan. Cook for 3-4 minutes, and then stir in the cauliflower rice. Clear a circle in the center of the pan and pour in the beaten eggs. Stir to scramble the eggs and then combine with the other ingredients. Season with salt and pepper to taste.

Notes
Servings: 2
Difficulty: Easy
⁇

139. Roasted Paleo Citrus and Herb Chicken

Ingredients

12 total pieces bone-in chicken thighs and legs

1 medium onion, thinly sliced

1 tbsp dried rosemary

1 tsp dried thyme

1 lemon, sliced thin

1 orange, sliced thin

For the marinade

5 tbsp extra virgin olive oil

6 cloves garlic, minced

1 tbsp honey

Juice of 1 lemon

Juice of 1 orange

1 tbsp Italian seasoning

1 tsp onion powder

Dash of red pepper flakes

Salt and freshly ground pepper, to taste

Instructions

Whisk together all of the marinade ingredients in a small bowl. Place the chicken in a baking dish (or a large Ziploc bag) and pour the marinade over it. Marinate for 3 hours to overnight.

Preheat the oven to 400 degrees F. Place the chicken in a baking dish and arrange with the onion, orange, and lemon slices. Sprinkle with thyme, rosemary, salt and pepper. Cover with aluminum foil and bake for 30 minutes. Remove the foil, baste the chicken, and bake for another 30 minutes uncovered, until the chicken is cooked through.

Notes

Servings: 4-6

Difficulty: Easy

[?]

140. Baked Sweet Potato Chips

Ingredients
2 large sweet potatoes
2 tbsp melted coconut oil
2 tsp dried rosemary
1 tsp sea salt

Instructions
Preheat oven to 375 degrees F. Peel sweet potatoes and slice thinly, using either a mandolin or sharp knife. In a large bowl, toss sweet potatoes with coconut oil, rosemary, and salt.
Place sweet potato chips in a single layer on a rimmed baking sheet covered with parchment paper. Bake in the oven for 10 minutes, then flip the chips over and bake for another 10 minutes. For the last ten minutes, watch the chips closely and pull off any chips that start to brown, until all of the chips are cooked.
⁇

141. Simple Baked Salmon with Lemon and Thyme

Ingredients
32 oz piece of salmon
1 lemon, sliced thin
1 tbsp capers
Salt and freshly ground pepper
1 tbsp fresh thyme
Olive oil, for drizzling

Instructions
Line a rimmed baking sheet with parchment paper and place salmon, skin side down, on the prepared baking sheet. Generously season salmon with salt and pepper. Arrange capers on the salmon, and top with sliced lemon and thyme.
Place baking sheet in a cold oven, then turn heat to 400 degrees F. Bake for 25 minutes. Serve immediately.
⁉

142. Refreshing Tomato Salsa Bowl Appetizer

Ingredients
4 medium ripe Roma tomatoes
1/4 cup black olives, sliced
1/4 cup onion, finely diced
1/2 green bell pepper, seeded and chopped
1/2 jalapeno, seeded and finely chopped
2 cloves garlic, minced
1 tbsp fresh cilantro, chopped
1 tbsp grapeseed oil
2 tsp balsamic vinegar
Salt and pepper, to taste

Instructions
Slice the tomatoes in half and scoop out the insides. In a small bowl, mix together the remaining ingredients. Stir well. Spoon the salsa mixture into the tomato cups. Serve chilled.

Notes
Servings: 4
Difficulty: Easy
?

143. Stove-top "Cheesy" Paleo Chicken Casserole

Ingredients
2 cups shredded cooked chicken
1 1/2 cups cooked butternut squash (about 1 small squash)
1/2 cup coconut cream, skimmed from the top of a can of coconut milk
1/4 cup coconut oil, melted
1 heaping cup green peas, thawed
1 tbsp apple cider vinegar
1/2 tsp salt
1/2 tsp oregano
1/2 tsp thyme
1 tbsp fresh parsley, for garnish

Instructions
In a large bowl, mash the butternut squash. Stir in the coconut cream, oil, vinegar, salt, oregano, and thyme. Once everything is combined, add in the shredded chicken and peas.
Place the mixture into a large saucepan and cook over medium heat for 5-8 minutes, until the peas are cooked and squash is creamy. Top with fresh parsley and serve warm.

Notes
Servings: 4-5
Difficulty: Medium
⏺

144. Asparagus Quiche with Spaghetti Squash Crust

Ingredients

1 medium spaghetti squash (use about 2 1/2 – 3 cups of the meat for this recipe)

2 tablespoons butter

1 large leek, thinly sliced

3 tablespoons butter

5 large eggs, beaten

1 cup coconut milk/almond milk/dairy milk (I used almond milk, as that's all that we had left)

a bunch of thin asparagus (about 2 cups), cut in halves or large pieces

1 medium tomato, cut in thin slices and then halve the slices

sea salt and freshly ground pepper, to taste

1/2 – 1 teaspoon ground nutmeg

Instructions

Preheat the oven to 375F (190C).

Carefully split the spaghetti squash in half. (It can also be baked whole, but it will take longer.)

Remove the seeds and sprouts, if any, with hands.

Place cut-side down on a baking pan.

Bake for 40 minutes, or until tender.

In the meantime, poach the asparagus in some water, until just tender. Remove from water and set aside.

Allow the spaghetti squash to cool a bit before removing the meat with a fork.

Mix about 2 1/2 to 3 cups of the meat with 2 tablespoons of butter and mix well.

Add sea salt and pepper, to taste. (Remember that the egg mixture will also contain seasoning, so don't go overboard.)

Pat the squash into a quiche form, covering the sides and bottom.

Bake at 400F (200C) for about 5-8 minutes, until golden and slightly crispy. Remove from oven and set aside.

In a saucepan, over medium heat, cook the leek slices with the 3 tablespoons butter, until tender.

Allow to slightly cool before pouring into the beaten eggs.

Add the milk, nutmeg, sea salt and pepper to taste.

Place the poached asparagus pieces on top of the spaghetti squash crust.

Pour the beaten eggs and leeks over top, covering the asparagus evenly.

Place the tomato pieces on top and bake for 35-40 minutes.

145. Garden Pea, Feta & Mint Tart

Garden Pea, Feta & Mint Tart (serves 6-8)

Crust:
1/2 cup butter, melted
2 large eggs
3/4 cup coconut flour
1/2 tsp sea salt

Instruction
Whisk together the eggs and butter.
Sieve the coconut flour into a large mixing bowl. Add the salt.
Gradually add the wet ingredients to the dry and mix until it forms a soft batter.
Press this into a greased 9in pie dish. It won't cooperate like regular dough, that's ok. Just press it in with your hands until the dish is covered. Prick the base.
Bake at 375 for 5 minutes. Remove and let cool while you sort out the filling.

Filling:
4oz feta cheese, crumbled
1 1/2 cups peas (I used frozen and defrosted beforehand)
2 spring/green onions, finely chopped
2 tbsps fresh mint leaves, chopped
3 large eggs
1/2 cup plain yoghurt
salt and pepper

Instructions
Whisk the eggs, yoghurt and seasoning together. Stir in the peas, feta and onions.
Fold in the mint and pour the whole mixture into your pie crust.
Bake at 375 for 25-30 mins till firm. Let cool for a few minutes before slicing up.
⁇

146. Garlicky Collard Pie

Ingredients

2 tablespoons ghee, butter or lard

1 small yellow onion, diced

4 cloves garlic, minced

4 cups collards or other hearty greens, rinsed and chopped

1 1/2 teaspoons kosher or sea salt

3/4 teaspoon freshly-ground black pepper

2 ounces pecorino romano or other hard Italian cheese, shredded

10 large eggs

3/4 cup coconut milk plus 1/2 cup water or 1 1/4 cups half and half

2 teaspoons garlic powder

1 teaspoon dried thyme

1 teaspoon dried oregano

Instructions

Preheat the oven to 375 F. Generously grease a 10" deep-dish pie plate with butter or non-hydrogenated palm oil shortening.

Melt the ghee in a large, heavy skillet over medium heat. Cook the onion until soft and almost translucent, about 5 minutes; add the garlic and cook for another minute more. Add the collard greens and cook, stirring frequently, until they are wilted. Season with the salt and pepper and remove from the heat.

In a large bowl, whisk together the eggs with the water, coconut milk, garlic powder, thyme and oregano until well blended. Spread the collard/onion mixture over the bottom of the greased pie plate; sprinkle the cheese evenly over the greens. Carefully pour the egg mixture over the cheese and greens.

Bake the pie for 25 to 35 minutes, or until the top is golden brown and a knife inserted in the center comes out clean.

Cool for 30 minutes before cutting into wedges. Serve with a chunky salsa or warm marinara sauce.

Nutrition (per serving): 203 calories, 15.5g total fat, 247.5mg cholesterol, 534.7mg sodium, 210.4mg potassium, 5.2g carbohydrates, 1.1g fiber, <1g sugar, 11.3g protein.

[?]

147. Crustless Broccoli and Sausage Quiche

Ingredients
1 medium onion, chopped
1 pound of bulk sausage (just remove casings if you can't find it in bulk)
2 cloves of garlic, grated
coconut oil
12 oz. of broccoli
10 eggs
sea salt/pepper/TJ's 21 seasoning salute

Instructions
Preheat your oven to 350 degrees. saute the onion in coconut oil over medium-highish heat. season with salt, pepper and 21 salute. once the onions are cooked halfway (translucent and soft) add the sausage meat. crumble the sausage as it cooks.

As the sausage is cooking, liberally grease a 9 x 13 pan in coconut oil. i suggest a small sandwich bag over your hand so you don't miss any spots or corners. next, in a large bowl, whisk the eggs vigorously. season with salt and pepper.

The broccoli i used was frozen in one of the steam-ready bags you throw into the microwave. instead of cooking it for 5 minutes in the microwave, i cooked it for only 2 so it was defrosted but not cooked all the way through. if you are using fresh broccoli, i would suggest blanching it for a minute or 2, any longer than that and it might get mushy. add the broccoli to the sausage mixture and cook for a minute or two.

Finally, add the garlic to the sausage mixture, cook for one additional minute and then remove from the heat. place the broccoli-sausage mixture into the greased baking dish. pour the eggs over the top of the meat and vegetables and bake uncovered for 25-30 minutes.

148. Crustless Mini Quiches

Ingredients
12 Large Omega 3 or other cage free, vegetarian fed, etc eggs
8 slices of bacon chopped and precooked
1 large carrot grated
1 large handful of spinach chopped finely
3 mini red bell peppers (or a couple tablespoons of a whole one), diced
3 mini yellow bell peppers (or part of a large one), diced
1/2 cup of chopped broccoli florets
2 green onions (or more if you like a strong onion flavour), chopped finely
1 chicken breast precooked with salt and pepper, diced (or any leftover meat, I just had this in the fridge)

Instructions
Preheat your oven to 350 degrees. Combine all of your ingredients and beat on high till frothy with electric mixer. Grease muffin tins with coconut oil liberally and pour in mixture 1/4 per muffin cup. Making sure to keep stirring up those goodies so they don't sink to the bottom while your filling your muffin cups. Bake at 350 degrees for about 20-25 minutes depending on your oven and muffin pans. Remove from oven and allow to cool for a few minutes, then run a knife around the edges to loosen, remove and eat warm or allow to cool completely to store for later.

These are a great grab and go breakfast or post WOD snack, make them ahead on the weekend and just warm up in the morning and go.

Post comments on your favourite versions to share with others. We would love to hear from you.
⍰

149.   Perfect Tomatillo Salsa Verde

Ingredients
1 lb. tomatillos, husked
1/2 medium onion, coarsely chopped
1 clove garlic, minced
1 Serrano pepper, seeded and coarsely chopped
1/4 cup fresh cilantro, chopped
Juice of 1/2 lime
1 tsp salt

Instructions
Place the tomatillos in a saucepan and cover with water. Broil to a boil, then turn the heat to simmer for 5 minutes. Remove with a slotted spoon.
Place the tomatillos and the remaining ingredients into a food processor and puree until smooth. Adjust salt to taste. Add water if necessary to reach desired consistency. Place in the refrigerator to chill before serving.

Notes
Servings: about 2 cups
Difficulty: Easy
⁇

150. Homemade Herbed Paleo Mayonnaise

Ingredients
1 egg (at room temperature)
2 tbsp lemon juice
1 tsp rosemary
1 tsp oregano
½ tsp sea salt
1 cup light olive oil (not EVOO – the flavour will be too strong)
This recipe will make approximately 24 1tbsp servings

Instructions
Add egg, lemon juice, rosemary, oregano, and sea salt to a mixing bowl.
Whisk together with an electric mixer on low until well blended. Don't turn off the mixer at any point during this process.
While still whisking, slowly add in your olive oil. Slow is the key word here. Like, one little drizzle at a time slow. Slowly but surely, you'll see the emulsion start to form. Once you see the emulsion forming, continue to add in your olive oil just as slowly until your mayonnaise reaches the desired consistency.
Refrigerate in a glass jar and enjoy! Will last in the fridge approximately one week.

Nutrition Facts Per Serving
Calories: 56
Total Fat: 6.5g
Saturated Fat: 1.0g
Carbs: 0.1g
Protein: 0.2g
⯑

151. Homemade Paleo Ketchup with a Kick

Ingredients

1 12 oz can tomato paste

1 cup water

2 tbsp vinegar

½ tsp salt

½ tsp curry powder

½ tsp garlic powder

This recipe makes approximately 32 oz of ketchup, or 64 1tbsp servings.

Instructions

Mix all ingredients in a sauce pan and bring to boil on medium-high heat.

Reduce heat to medium-low and simmer while stirring frequently until flavours have blended. (Add more water for thinner ketchup, add less water for thicker)

Transfer to a glass jar and cool before serving.

Nutrition Facts Per Serving

Calories: 5

Total Fat: 0.0g

Sodium: 21mg

Carbs: 1.0g

Protein: 0.7g

⏎

152.   Homemade Paleo Honey Mustard from Scratch

Ingredients
1/4 cup mustard powder
1/4 cup water
3 tbsp honey
Sea salt, to taste

Instructions
Place the mustard powder and water in a bowl and stir until combined. Add salt and honey to taste. Let stand for at least 15 minutes before serving.

Notes
Servings: about 1/2 cup
Difficulty: Easy
⁇

153. All-Natural Homemade Paleo Apple Butter

Ingredients
5 apples, peeled, cored and diced
2/3 cup apple cider
1/3 cup honey
1 tbsp cinnamon
1/2 tsp salt
Pinch of cloves, optional

Instructions
Place all of the ingredients into the slow cooker and stir to evenly coat. Cover and cook on low heat for 6 hours. Let cool slightly and puree in a food processor or blender until smooth.

Notes
Servings: 4-6
Difficulty: Easy
⁇

154. Fresh and Easy Arugula Pesto

Ingredients
2 cups fresh arugula, packed
1/4 cup walnuts
2 cloves garlic, peeled
1/2 tsp lemon juice
1/2 tsp salt
1/2 cup extra virgin olive oil

Instructions
Add the arugula, walnuts, garlic, lemon juice, and salt to a blender or food processor and blend. Gradually add the olive oil and process until well combined.

Notes
Servings: about 2/3 cup
Difficulty: Easy
⏺

155. Homemade Paleo BBQ Sauce (YUM)

Ingredients
15 oz. organic tomato sauce
1 cup water
1/2 cup apple cider vinegar
1/3 cup honey
1 tbsp lemon juice
2 tsp onion powder
1 1/2 tsp ground black pepper
1 1/2 tsp ground mustard
1 tsp paprika

Instructions
Combine all of the ingredients in a medium saucepan over medium-high heat. Stir to combine. Bring to a boil, and then reduce to simmer for 1 hour. Taste and adjust seasonings as desired. Serve with meat or store in an airtight container in the refrigerator.

Notes
Servings: about 1 1/2 cups
Difficulty: Easy
⏎

156. Basil Pesto

Ingredients
1 large bunch of basil (approx. 2 cups)
1/3 cup walnuts or pine nuts
2 medium garlic cloves, minced
1/2 cup Parmigiano Reggiano or other Parmesan cheese (optional)
approx. 1/3 cup extra virgin olive oil
salt and pepper to taste

Instructions
Place basil, nuts, garlic and cheese (optional) in food processor.
Run the food processor, pausing to add olive oil to reach desired consistency.
Salt and pepper to taste.
🔲

157. Radicchio Pesto

Serves 4
Ingredients
1 radicchio head, roughly chopped (ribs and leaves)
3 tablespoons grated Romano cheese
3 tablespoons grated Parmesan cheese
⅓ cup / 1.8 oz / 50 gr blanched almonds
tablespoons warm water, plus more if needed
½ teaspoon fine grain sea salt
Ground black pepper to taste
2 tablespoons olive oil

Instructions
Place the cut radicchio in a small bowl of cold water and allow to sit for 30 minutes. This will remove some of the bitterness. Drain and squeeze out as much water as possible. (Note: you can skip this step if you're in a hurry).
Heat a skillet over medium heat. Add almonds and toast for 5 minutes. Set aside.
In a food processor add (toasted) almonds; pulse until the mixture resembles a coarse meal.
Add the radicchio and 2 tablespoons of water.
Pulse until the radicchio is broken up and nearly smooth.
Using a spatula, scrape down the sides.
Add Parmesan cheese, Romano cheese, salt and pepper. Pulse again and while the food processor is running slowly add the water - one tablespoon at a time - until the pesto reaches a creamy consistency.
Transfer radicchio pesto to a bowl and using a spoon stir in the olive oil until it's completely absorbed.
If the pesto looks too thick, add more olive oil (or water), one tablespoon   at a time until it reaches the desired consistency.

Nutrition facts
One serving yields 165 calories, 15 grams of fat, 3 grams of carbs and 6 grams of protein
⍰

158.   Herbed Calamari Salad with Preserved Lemons

Ingredients

3 Tablespoons extra virgin olive oil

2 to 3 medium cloves garlic, smashed and minced

2 1/2 pounds cleaned and trimmed uncooked calamari rings and tentacles (defrosted)

3/4 teaspoon kosher salt

1/4 teaspoon freshly ground black pepper

pinch crushed red pepper flakes

juice of 1 large lemon

1/4 cup finely chopped mint leaves

1/4 cup finely chopped cilantro leaves

1/2 cup finely chopped flat-leaf parsley leaves

peel of 1 preserved lemon, thinly sliced

Instructions

Begin by defrosting the calamari (if purchased frozen). Place in a strainer and run under cold water for 15 to 20 minutes, tossing a couple of times, until soft and pliable. Drain water, pat dry with paper towels and set aside.

Use a paring knife to remove just the rind from the preserved lemon. Discard the inside and thinly slice the rind.

Smash garlic and mince. Finely chop cleaned mint, cilantro and parsley.

COOK:

Heat a very large skillet or frying pan over medium high heat. Once hot, add 1 1/2 Tablespoons of olive oil. Heat oil and add garlic.

Saute, stirring constantly, for 20 to 30 seconds until fragrant and add in defrosted and well-drained calamari (If your pan isn't large enough to accommodate all the calamari in one layer, divide the 1 1/2 T olive oil and cook the calamari in batches. You do not want them to steam, you want them to sear and for that, they must cook in a single layer with some room around them).Sprinkle with a pinch of salt and pepper and continue cooking for 2 to 4 minutes or until opaque and just firm. You do not want to overcook the calamari or it be have a rubbery texture.

Drain off any liquid that is released during cooking and remove cooked calamari to a mixing bowl.

Add remaining 1 1/2 Tablespoons olive oil, salt, pepper, red pepper flakes, lemon juice, preserved lemon rind and herbs to mixing bowl and toss well while calamari still warm.

Adjust seasoning if necessary, cover and chill until ready to serve. This is nice served over some spring greens or other delicate lettuce with some ripe cucumbers or grape tomatoes. Enjoy!

159. Legendary Gluten-Free Blueberry Crisp (YUM!)

Ingredients
2 pints fresh blueberries
Juice of 1 lemon
1 cup almond flour
1/2 cup slivered almonds
1/4 cup coconut oil, melted
2 tbsp maple syrup
1 tsp cinnamon
1/8 tsp salt
Pinch of nutmeg

Instructions
Preheat the oven to 375 degrees F. In a small bowl, toss the blueberries with the lemon juice. Divide between six ramekin dishes.
Using the same bowl, mix together the remaining ingredients until combined. Spoon the almond crumble over the blueberries. Bake for 30-35 minutes, until bubbly and golden brown. Let cool slightly before serving.

Notes
Servings: 6 ramekins
Difficulty: Easy
⬚

160. Paleo Chicken Tortilla Soup

Ingredients
2 large chicken breasts, skin removed and cut into ½ inch strips
1 28oz can of diced tomatoes
32 ounces organic chicken broth
1 sweet onion, diced
2 jalepenos, de-seeded and diced
2 cups of shredded carrots
2 cups chopped celery
1 bunch of cilantro chopped fine
4 cloves of garlic, minced - I always use one of these
2 Tbs tomato paste
1 tsp chili powder
1 tsp cumin
sea salt & fresh cracked pepper to taste
olive oil
1-2 cups water

Instructions
In a crockpot or large dutch oven over med-high heat, place a dash of olive oil and about ¼ cup chicken broth. Add onions, garlic, jalapeno, sea salt and pepper and cook until soft, adding more broth as needed. Then add all of your remaining ingredients and enough water to fill to the top of your pot. Cover and let cook on low for about 2 hrs, adjusting salt & pepper as needed.
Once the chicken is fully cooked, you should be able to shred it very easily. I simply used the back of a wooden spoon and pressed the cooked chicken against the side of the pot. You could also use a fork or tongs to break the chicken apart and into shreds.
Top with avocado slices and fresh cilantro. Enjoy!
This is an easy one-pot meal that's loaded with veggies, low in fat, and full of flavour! You don't need to add cheese or tortilla strips the soup is full of flavour on its own!
?

161. Butternut Squash & Kale Beef Stew

Ingredients
2 tbsp bacon fat, or cooking oil of choice
2 lb stew beef, 1" cubed
1 onion, roughly chopped
4 garlic cloves, minced
1 1/2 tbsp fresh sage, minced
1/2 tsp smoked paprika
1 small butternut squash, cubed (about 4 cups)
16oz frozen, chopped kale (or one bunch fresh)
4 cups beef stock, preferably homemade
salt and pepper

Instructions
In a large dutch oven heat 1 tbsp bacon fat over medium high. Working in batches, brown the meat, making sure not to cook it through (it can turn tough).
Set browned meat aside. Lower heat to medium and add the 2nd tbsp bacon fat. Once it's melted add the onions, garlic, smoked paprika, and sage to pot, along with a big pinch of salt and fresh pepper. Cook about 8 minutes, or until the onions begin to soften and turn translucent. Make sure to stir frequently so the mixture doesn't burn.
Add the beef, butternut squash, and kale to the pot. Stir to combine, then add the chicken stock and two cups of hot water. Bring to a boil, then reduce to a simmer and let cook, covered, for at least an hour. I let mine go about 45 minutes longer.
⁇

162. Bacon and Tomato Quiche

Ingredients
Zucchini Hash Crust:
2 small to medium size organic zucchini, grated
1 egg, beaten
1 1/2 Tbsp coconut flour
1 tsp flax meal *optional
1 tbsp butter or coconut oil melted
1/8 tsp sea salt

Quiche:
5 eggs, beaten
1/2 cup organic egg whites, (I used the ones in a carton, but make sure egg white is the only ingredient) or you could separate 3 eggs
3 Tbsp milk of choice: organic heavy cream, or unsweetened plain almond milk
5 slices nitrate free bacon, cooked and chopped (make sure bacon has no sugar in the ingredients)
2/3 cup cauliflower, ground into rice (you won't taste it, and it adds nutrients and fiber)
1/2 cup fresh spinach, chopped * optional
1/4 tsp ground mustard
1/4 tsp sea salt (I use Real Salt or Himalayan sea salt)
1/4 tsp black pepper

Topping:
2 small to medium sized tomatoes, sliced (I used 6 slices).
1/2 cup grated cheese of choice * optional

Instructions
Preheat oven to 400 F, and grease or oil pie dish.
Grate or use processor on zucchini.
Wrap grated zucchini in layered paper towels or cheese cloth. Squeeze and drain liquid from zucchini over sink. Place drained zucchini in large bowl.
Add all the remaining crust ingredients to the zucchini and mix together.
Place zucchini mixture into pie dish. Use the back of a spoon to spread mixture around pie dish, until dish is covered in zucchini crust mixture.
Bake zucchini crust in oven for 9 minutes.

Remove crust from oven (leave oven on). Set aside.

In large mixing bowl combine: eggs, egg whites, milk of choice, ground mustard, sea salt, and black pepper.

Grate or use processor on the cauliflower until rice texture forms.

Add cauliflower rice, chopped spinach, and chopped bacon to the egg mixture and combine.

Pour egg mixture into zucchini crust.

Place tomato slices on top of quiche.

Bake for 28 minutes, but check at 20 minutes to see if crust edges are browning too much.

Loosely cover the top of pie dish with a parchment paper sheet. Place back in oven for remaining 8 minutes, or until top is browned and center is firm and set.

Add optional cheese and put back in oven for 2 minutes.

Remove and let cool.

Slice and serve.

Notes

Net Carb Count*: 8.15 g net carbs (per 1 slice - makes 8 slices)

Total Carb Count: 11.79 g total carbs (per 1 slice - makes 8 slices)

▢

163.   Paleo Eggs Benedict on Artichoke Hearts

Ingredients
4 eggs
1 egg white (use from Hollandaise Sauce Recipe below)
250 grams of bacon
4 Artichoke Hearts
3/4 cup of balsamic vinegar
salt and pepper to taste
Hollandaise Sauce
4 egg yolks
1 tbsp of lemon juice
pinch of salt and paprika
¾ cup of melted ghee

Instructions
Line a baking sheet with foil and set aside. Preheat your oven to 375 degrees. Deconstruct your artichokes and remove the artichoke hearts. Place the hearts in balsamic vinegar for 20 minutes.
For your Hollandaise Sauce, place a pot of water to simmer on your stove. Melt the ghee in a saucepan. Separate your eggs and place the yolks in a stainless steel cooking bowl. Hold on to the egg whites for the next step.
Remove your hearts from the marinade and place on cookie sheet, brush the tops of them with the egg white and then place your bacon over the artichokes as a second layer. Stick your tray in the oven for 20 minutes.
Back to the sauce, whisk the yolks with the lemon juice and then place your bowl over the simmering water. Slowly add in the ghee and bit of salt and continue to whisk until your sauce doubles in size and is silky. Set aside.
To poach your eggs, turn up the heat on your stove and let the same water get to a rolling boil. Crack your eggs one at a time into a ladle and the slide the egg into the water. Give them about a minute and a half and remove.
Now you are ready to assemble. Grab your artichoke hearts and bacon, then lay your poached egg and pour the Hollandaise silk on top.
⏹

164. Hearty Paleo Jambalaya

Ingredients
1 tbsp extra virgin olive oil
8 oz. Andouille sausage, diced
1/2 red bell pepper, diced
1/2 yellow bell pepper, diced
4 cloves garlic, minced
1/2 medium onion, diced
1 14.5-oz. can fire-roasted tomatoes
1 tbsp smoked paprika
1 tsp dried thyme
1 tsp cumin
Dash of cayenne pepper
1 1/2 cups chicken broth
1 large head of cauliflower, coarsely chopped
1 lb. medium shrimp, peeled and deveined
Salt and pepper, to taste
Fresh cilantro, for garnish

Instructions
Heat the olive oil in a Dutch oven or heavy-bottomed saucepan. Add the Andouille sausages and cook for 4-5 minutes until lightly browned. Add the red and yellow peppers, garlic, and onion and stir. Cook for 4 minutes until softened.
Stir in the tomatoes and spices. Pour in the chicken stock and bring to a boil. Once boiling, turn the heat down and simmer for 20 minutes.
Meanwhile, place the cauliflower into a food processor and pulse until it is reduced to the size of rice grains.
Mix in the cauliflower rice to the jambalaya, starting with half of the rice and adding more depending on preference. Simmer for 12-15 minutes until tender. Add the shrimp and cook everything for 5-7 minutes until the shrimp are opaque. Season to taste with salt and pepper. Serve hot, garnished with fresh cilantro.

Notes
Servings: 4-6
Difficulty: Easy

?

165.   Shrimp & Grits (Paleo Style)

Ingredients

For the shrim:

15 pieces raw shrimp, shelled and de-veined

3 tbsp extra virgin olive oil

6 garlic cloves minced, divided

Zest from one lemon

2 tsp dried oregano, divided

2 slices bacon

1/2 large onion, diced

2 tbsp butter

1 tbsp white wine vinegar

1 tsp red pepper flakes

1 tbsp lemon juice

1 tbsp chopped fresh oregano

Salt and freshly ground black pepper, to taste

For the grit:

1 large head of cauliflower, cut into florets

1/4 cup almond milk

4 garlic cloves, minced

1 tbsp ghee or butter

1/4 tsp cayenne pepper

Salt and pepper, to taste

Instructions

In a medium bowl mix together the olive oil, 2 cloves of garlic, lemon zest, and 1 teaspoon dried oregano. Place shrimp in the bowl and marinate for 1-3 hours.

Place a couple inches of water in a large pot. Once water is boiling, place steamer insert and then cauliflower florets into the pot and cover. Steam for 12-14 minutes, until completely tender. Drain and return cauliflower to pot.

Add the milk, ghee, and garlic to the cauliflower. Using an immersion blender, combine ingredients. The cauliflower should be fairly thick to resemble the consistency of grits. Season with salt and pepper to taste.

Cook the bacon in a large skillet over medium heat until crispy. Reserving the bacon fat in the pan, set the bacon aside to cool and break into pieces.

Add the butter to the bacon fat in the pan and melt. Add the onion and sauté for 4-5 minutes until softened. Add in the remaining 4 garlic cloves, dried oregano, and the red pepper flakes. Sauté for 1-2 minutes, stirring frequently.

Stir in the white wine vinegar, and then add the shrimp. Cook, stirring frequently, until the shrimp are cooked through, 3-4 minutes. Remove from heat and stir in the lemon juice. Season with salt and pepper. Serve shrimp and onions over grits, with bacon and fresh oregano for garnish.

Notes
Servings: 3-4
Difficulty: Medium

166. Paleo Turkey Pesto Meatballs

Ingredients
2 lbs. ground turkey
1/2 cup almond flour
1/2 cup pesto
2 egg whites
1/2 tsp salt
1/4 tsp freshly ground pepper

Instructions
Preheat the oven to 375 degrees F. Line a baking sheet with aluminum foil and then place a wire cooling rack on top of the baking sheet. Coat the wire rack well with coconut oil spray.
In a large bowl, mix together all of the ingredients. Roll the mixture into small balls using your hands and place on the wire rack. Bake for 20-25 minutes until cooked through.

Notes
Servings: 24 meatballs
Difficulty: Easy
🔲

167.   Broccoli Egg Bake (So Wholesome & Healthy)

Ingredients
8 eggs
1/2 large onion, diced
2 medium zucchini, diced
1 medium head of broccoli, chopped
1 tsp salt
1/2 tsp freshly ground black pepper
1 tbsp fresh parsley, chopped

Instructions
Preheat the oven to 350 degrees F. In a small bowl, whisk the eggs, salt and pepper. Stir in the chopped vegetables.
Grease a ramekin with coconut oil spray. Pour egg mixture into the dish and bake for 25-30 minutes or until the eggs are set. Remove from heat and let sit for 5 minutes before serving. Top with chopped parsley to serve.

Notes
Servings: 6
Difficulty: Easy
⁇

168. Meatball Sandwich with Zucchini "Bread" & Coconut Curry Sauce

Ingredients
Meatball:
½ onion
½ tomato
4 cloves of garlic
1 egg
2 tbsp coconut milk
2 tsp sea salt
½ tsp black pepper
½ tsp paprika
1 lb. of grass-fed ground beef.
Zucchini "bread" and coconut sauce
1 onion
1 tomato
3 cloves of garlic
250g can coconut milk
4 very large zucchinis or 8 small ones (one per sandwich)
1 tsp sea salt
1 tsp curry powder
1 lemon
Parsley

Instructions
Preheat your over to 350 degrees. Line two roasting trays with aluminum foil.
Dice your tomato, onion and garlic. Set aside.
For the meatballs, crack open your egg and mix in tomato, onion, garlic, salt, black pepper and coconut milk.
It's time to get intimate with your creation. Put your beef into a mixing bowl and using your hands knead in the egg mixture. Shape into lovely little meatballs and place on roasting tray and put tray into heated oven for 20 minutes.
While your meatballs form into edible creations take your washed zucchini and slice them in half. Then dig out about 1/3 of the zucchini meat on one half and ½ from the top half.

Dice up the zucchini meat and add onion, tomato, garlic, salt, curry powder and add the coconut cream only (the water on the bottom is not needed so use it tomorrow for a tasty addition to a Crockpot chicken soup).

Mix everything and pour into your waiting zucchini tunnels. Remove your meatballs from the oven and place your zucchini into the oven at the same temperature.

Cook your guys for 20 minutes uncovered and then cover them with a sheet of foil for another 10 minutes. Chop up your parsley and lemon wedges for plating.

Remove zucchini from oven and sprinkle some lemon juice on top. Nestle the meatballs into the deeper zucchini half place your second zucchini half on top, slice in half and serve with some parsley and lemon on the side for a mini salad garnish.

Notes

You can use a knife and fork but for sandwich-style eating wrap the bottom halves of your sandwiches in wax paper (the red and white checkered kind if you can get it) so you can hold on to your grub and have a delightful conversation at the same time.

⁇

169. Easy Homemade Gluten-Free Energy Bars

Ingredients
1 cup almonds
1 cup dried cranberries
1 cup pitted dates
1 tbsp unsweetened coconut flakes
1/4 cup mini dark chocolate chips

Instructions
Combine all of the ingredients in a blender or food processor. Pulse a few times to break everything up. Then blend continuously until the ingredients have broken down and start to clump together into a ball. Using a spatula to scrape down the sides, turn out the mixture onto a piece of wax paper or plastic wrap. Press into an even square and chill, wrapped, for at least an hour. Cut into desired size of bars, wrapping each bar in plastic wrap to store in the fridge.

Notes
Servings: 8 bars
Difficulty: Easy
⯑

170. How to Make Paleo Cauliflower "Rice"

Ingredients
1 head of cauliflower
½ Vidalia onion
3 cloves of garlic
1 tbsp coconut oil
salt and pepper, to taste
This recipe makes 2-3 servings, depending on the size of your cauliflower.

Instructions
Remove leaves and stem from cauliflower; discard. Grate the entire head of cauliflower until it resembles rice.
Dice the onions and garlic to your desired size.
Add coconut oil to a pan over medium heat. Add in onion and garlic until slightly browned.
Add in grated cauliflower, salt, and pepper and stir until heated.
⁇

SNACKS

171. Addictive & Healthy Paleo Nachos

Ingredients

2 medium tomatoes, diced and seeded

2 tbsp fresh cilantro, chopped

1-2 tbsp lime juice

2 cups guacamole

2 tbsp green onions, chopped

For the sweet potato chips

3 large sweet potatoes

3 tbsp melted coconut oil

1 tsp salt

For the meat

1 medium yellow onion, finely diced

1 tbsp coconut oil

1 green chili, diced

1 lb. ground beef

2 cloves garlic, minced

1 tsp smoked paprika

1/2 tsp ground cumin

1 tbsp tomato paste

12 oz. canned diced tomatoes

1 tsp salt

1/2 tsp pepper

Instructions

To make the sweet potato chips, preheat the oven to 375 degrees F. Peel the sweet potatoes and slice thinly, using either a mandolin or sharp knife. In a large bowl, toss them with coconut oil and salt. Place the chips in a single layer on a rimmed baking sheet covered with parchment paper. Bake in the oven for 10 minutes, then flip the chips over and bake for another 10 minutes. For the last ten minutes, watch the chips closely and pull off any chips that start to brown, until all of the chips are cooked.

While the potato chips are baking, start preparing the beef. Melt the coconut oil in a large skillet over medium heat. Add the onion and chili to the pan and sauté for 3-4 minutes until softened. Add the ground beef and cook for 4-5 minutes, stirring regularly. Add the garlic, diced tomatoes, tomato paste, and remaining spices and stir well to combine. Bring the mixture to a simmer and then turn the heat down to medium-low. Cook, covered, for 20-25 minutes, stirring regularly.

Stir the chopped tomatoes, lime juice, and cilantro into the beef mixture. Adjust salt and pepper to taste. Remove from heat.

To assemble the nachos, form a large circle with the sweet potato chips on a platter. Add the beef mixture into the middle of the circle, and then top with guacamole and green onions.

Notes
Servings: 4-6
Difficulty: Medium

172. Homemade Paleo Tortilla Chips

Ingredients
1 cup almond flour
1 egg white
1/2 tsp salt
1/2 tsp chili powder
1/2 tsp garlic powder
1/2 tsp cumin
1/4 tsp onion powder
1/4 tsp paprika

Instructions
Preheat the oven to 325 degrees F. In a large bowl, combine all of the ingredients together until they form an even dough.
Roll out the dough between two pieces of parchment paper, as thinly as possible. Remove the top layer of parchment paper. Cut the dough into desired shapes for chips.
Move the dough, with the parchment paper, onto a baking sheet. Bake for 11-13 minutes, until golden brown.
Remove from the oven and let cool 5 minutes. Use a spatula to remove the chips from the paper. Serve with guacamole or salsa.
🔲

173. Paleo Chocolate Cookies (I Can't Get Enough of These)

Ingredients
2 tbsp and 2 tsp coconut oil
3 oz. unsweetened dark chocolate
1/4 cup honey
2 eggs
1 1/2 tsp vanilla extract
1/2 cup coconut flour
1/2 tsp cinnamon

Instructions
In a large microwave-safe bowl, melt the coconut oil and chocolate in the microwave, stirring intermittently. Let cool for 5 minutes.
Add the eggs, vanilla, and honey to the chocolate mixture. Stir well to make sure not to scramble the eggs.
Add in the coconut flour and cinnamon and mix well. Place in the refrigerator for approximately 30 minutes, until slightly hardened.
Preheat oven to 350 degrees F. Roll out the dough between two pieces of parchment paper until 1/4-inch thick. Cut out shapes with a cookie cutter and carefully place on a parchment-lined baking sheet. Repeat this step for remaining dough.
Bake cookies for 12-15 minutes. Allow to cool before serving.

Notes
Servings: approximately 18 cookies
Difficulty: Medium
⁇

174. Easy Paleo Shepherd's Pie

Ingredients
For the top layer
1 large head cauliflower, cut into florets
2 tbsp ghee, melted
1 tsp spicy Paleo mustard
Salt and freshly ground black pepper, to taste
Fresh parsley, to garnish

For the bottom layer
1 tbsp coconut oil
1/2 large onion, diced
3 carrots, diced
2 celery stalks, diced
1 lb. lean ground beef
2 tbsp tomato paste
1 cup chicken broth
1 tsp dry mustard
1/4 tsp cinnamon
1/8 tsp ground clove
Salt and freshly ground black pepper, to taste

Instructions
Place a couple inches of water in a large pot. Once the water is boiling, place steamer insert and then cauliflower florets into the pot and cover. Steam for 12-14 minutes, until tender. Drain and return cauliflower to the pot.
Add the ghee, mustard, salt, and pepper to the cauliflower. Using an immersion blender or food processor, combine the ingredients until smooth. Set aside.
Meanwhile, heat the coconut oil in a large skillet over medium heat. Add the onion, celery, and carrots and sauté for 5 minutes. Add in the ground beef and cook until browned.
Stir the tomato paste, chicken broth, and remaining spices into the meat mixture. Season to taste with salt and pepper. Simmer until most of the liquid has evaporated, about 8 minutes, stirring occasionally.
Distribute the meat mixture evenly among four ramekins and spread the pureed cauliflower on top. Use a fork to create texture in the cauliflower and drizzle with olive oil. Place under the broiler for 5-7 minutes until the top turns golden. Sprinkle with fresh parsley and serve.

Notes
Servings: 4
Difficulty: Medium

175. Spicy Avocado Dill Dressing

Ingredients
1 very ripe avocado
2 tablespoons olive oil
3 sprigs fresh dill
1 tbsp chili powder (more or less to taste)
1 tbsp lime juice
1 tbsp honey
2 tbsp apple cider vinegar
2 cloves garlic
¼ cup almond milk
¼ cup water

Instructions
Combine all ingredients in a blender, process until creamy.
Store in an airtight jar or container in refrigerator, will last approximately 1 week.

Nutrition Facts per serving
Calories: 104
Fat: 9.2g
Saturated Fat: 2.7g
Carbs: 6.3g
Fiber: 2.4g
Protein: 1.1g
⁂

176. No-Bake Walnut Cookies (Grain-Free & Gluten-Free)

Ingredients
1 cup walnuts
1/2 cup unsweetened coconut flakes
2 tbsp raw honey
1/2 tsp vanilla extract
1/4 tsp salt

Instructions
Add walnuts to food processor and blend until finely ground. Add in the remaining ingredients and blend until a dough forms, about a minute.
Turn out the dough onto a piece of parchment paper. Using your hands, roll pieces of the dough into small balls, about 1 inch around, and space out on parchment paper. After all of the balls are formed, press down on each ball to form a flat cookie. Place in the freezer for at least 30 minutes before serving. Store in an airtight container in the freezer.

Notes
Servings: Makes 10-12 cookies
Difficulty: Easy
⁇

177. Paleo French Toast with Blueberry Syrup

Ingredients
1 loaf Paleo bread (I used this recipe for Paleo Bread)
1/2 cup almond milk
2 eggs
1/2 tbsp vanilla
1 tsp cinnamon

Instructions
In a large bowl, whisk together the coconut milk, eggs, vanilla and cinnamon.
Heat a griddle or non-stick skillet to medium-high. Coat pan with coconut oil. Dip a slice of bread into the batter mixture to coat both sides, letting any excess drip off. Place the bread onto the pan and cook each side until slightly browned. Repeat with remaining bread. Serve warm.

Notes
Servings: 4
Difficulty: Easy
⬚

178. Lavender Maca Brownies (Dairy & Grain Free)

Ingredients
1/3 cup water
1/3 cup extra virgin olive oil
2 eggs
1 ½ cups almond flour
1 teaspoon baking powder
1 teaspoon salt
2/3 cup unsweetened cocoa powder
1 cup honey (I like to use raw honey found at my local farmer's market)
¾ cup semisweet chocolate chips
1 tablespoon dried lavender flowers (having a few left over for decoration)
1 tablespoon maca powder
Himalayan pink salt (optional)

Instructions
Preheat oven to 350 degrees F and grease a 9x13" baking pan. (Brownies made in this size pan will be about one inch thick once baked – if you want them fuller, use a smaller sized pan)
Whisk together the water, olive oil, and eggs in a large bowl.
Slowly whisk in the flour, baking powder, salt, honey, maca powder, and cocoa powder one ingredient at a time. If you're using raw honey and it's too thick to whisk in, melt it in the microwave for about 20 seconds before adding it to your batter.
Once the batter is well blended, add in your lavender and chocolate chips. The measurement for the lavender is up to you – I found one tablespoon to be the perfect amount, but depending on how floral you want these brownies to be you could add more or less.
Pour the batter into a baking pan and spread until it is in one even layer. Don't worry if the batter seems too thick, that's how it's supposed to be.
Bake for about 20 minutes, until a toothpick inserted in the center comes out clean.
Let cool, then sprinkle fresh lavender and Himalayan pink salt over the top before cutting.
Enjoy the fruits of your labor!!

Notes
This recipe should make approximately 24 2x2" square brownies.
⬚

179. The Best Paleo Brownies (Chocolaty Goodness)

Ingredients
1 cup paleo-friendly almond butter
1/3 cup maple syrup
1 egg
2 tbsp ghee
1 tsp vanilla
1/3 cup cocoa powder
1/2 tsp baking soda

Instructions
Preheat the oven to 325 degrees F. In a large bowl, whisk together the almond butter, syrup, egg, ghee, and vanilla. Stir in the cocoa powder and baking soda.
Pour the batter into a 9-inch baking pan. Bake for 20-23 minutes, until the brownie is done, but still soft in the middle.

Notes
Servings: 6
Difficulty: Easy
⬜

180. Homemade Baked Cinnamon Apple Chips

Ingredients
1-2 apples (I used Honeycrisp)
1 tsp cinnamon

Instructions
Preheat oven to 200 degrees.
Using a sharp knife or mandolin, slice apples thinly. Discard seeds. Prepare a baking sheet with parchment paper and arrange apple slices on it without overlapping.
Sprinkle cinnamon over apples.
Bake for approximately 1 hour, then flip. Continue baking for 1-2 hours, flipping occasionally, until the apple slices are no longer moist. Store in airtight container.
⁇

DESSERTS

181. Paleo Antioxidant Berry Shake

Ingredients
1/2 cup coconut milk
1/4 cup cold water
1/2 frozen banana
1/2 cup frozen raspberries
1/2 cup frozen blueberries
1 tbsp chia seeds

Instructions
In a large cup (if using an immersion blender) or a blender, combine ingredients and blend until smooth. Add more water if necessary to reach desired consistency. Serve immediately.

Notes
Servings: 1
Difficulty: Easy
⬚

182. Paleo Pumpkin Pie Smoothie

Ingredients

1 frozen banana

2 tbsp pumpkin puree

½ cup unsweetened almond milk

½ tsp vanilla extract

1 tsp honey

1 tbsp hemp hearts

¼ tsp cinnamon

¼ tsp cloves

¼ tsp nutmeg

Instructions

Combine all ingredients in a blender and process until smooth. I find it's easier on the blender if I break the frozen banana into smaller chunks before processing.

Pour into a tall glass and enjoy with your favourite book, your favourite music, or both!

Notes

Calories: 220

Total Fat: 6.4g

Saturated Fat: 0.8g

Carbs: 38.0g

Fiber: 6.1g

Protein: 5.6g

⏹

183. Green Kale Smoothie with Mango

Ingredients
2 large leaves of kale
2 frozen bananas (peeled and cut into thirds)
1 frozen mango (diced)
2 tablespoons maca powder
2 tablespoons hemp hearts
3 cups unsweetened almond milk
This recipe makes two large smoothies, can be halved for one serving.

Instructions
Add frozen banana chunks and frozen mango chunks into a blender with the almond milk. Blend until smooth. (I freeze my fruit in chunks to make it easier on the blender)
Add in kale, maca powder, and hemp hearts. Blend until smooth.
Serve immediately and enjoy!!

Nutrition Facts (per smoothie)
Calories: 294
Fat: 9.0g
Saturated fat: 0.7g
Sodium: 274mg
Carbs: 51.0g
Fiber: 8.6g
Protein: 7.7g
⑦

184. Healthy Fruit Leather

Ingredients
2 apples, finely diced
10 strawberries, diced
1 ruby pink grapefruit, diced
Stevia/rice malt syrup to sweeten if needed
1 tsp cinnamon
Pinch salt
1/4 cup water

Instructions
Place the fruit in saucepan with the water and bring to a boil. Reduce the heat and simmer until the fruit is soft and the liquid has been reduced. Stir through the cinnamon and salt.
Transfer the fruit to a blender and puree until smooth. Taste the mixture and if required add a sweetener. The grapefruit can be quite tart and while suitable for adults children may not appreciate this. If you would like a sweeter roll up than I suggest adding some sweetness to balance out the sourness. If a sweetener is added blend again until combined. You should end up with 2-3 cups worth of pureed fruit. Heat oven to 120-150°C (250-300F). Line a large baking tray with baking paper (if your baking tray is not very large you may need to use two smaller sized trays).
Pour the mixture onto the tray and spread it out thinly by using the back of a spatula. You want it to just cover the baking paper's surface without leaving any gaps (the thinner the better!). Place the baking tray in the oven on the lowest shelf available and bake for 8-12 hours. I left mine overnight baking at about 130°C for 9 hours. Remove the tray from the oven and using a sharp knife cut the fruit leather into strips. Let it cool completely before peeling the fruit leather off the baking paper. Roll up if desired and store in an airtight container for up to a week! Enjoy :)
⁂

185. Gummi Orange Slices

Ingredients
1 T. vanilla extract
½ t. natural orange flavour
Pinch real salt
1 ½ t. liquid stevia (every brand varies in sweetness, so add this 'to taste')
8 T. grass-fed gelatin
1 can coconut milk
1 ½ C. water
Natural orange food colouring to desired colour
orange ice cube tray molds

Instructions
Heat water and coconut milk over low heat until simmering.
Continue on low heat, slowly adding in each tablespoon of gelatin, whisking the entire time.
Add remaining ingredients and whisk until any clumps of gelatin are gone.
Pour into molds, and pour remaining liquid into 8X8 glass pan.
Put in fridge until solid. Gummis should pop out easily once hardened.
☐

186. Prosciutto-Wrapped Berries

Yields: 12 total strawberries/baby bell peppers

Ingredients

6 strawberries

6 golden baby bell peppers

Honey Basil Ricotta (see below)

1 oz. thinly sliced grass-fed proscuitto, divided into 12 strips

1/4 c. micro greens (about half a small package)

Instructions

Using a sharp pairing knife, cut the tops off the strawberries, pulling the middle completely out and leaving a deep hole. Do the same for the peppers and use your finger to pull any seeds out of the insides. To assemble: use a butter knife to stuff the berries/peppers with about 1 t. each of the Honey Basil Ricotta (the peppers will hold more ricotta than the berries). Then place a few sprigs of micro greens into the ricotta.

Wrap a thin slice of proscuitto around each one and lay down length-wise to hold the proscuitto in place (you could also use toothpicks for this but that's a little too fussy for me).

⏷

187. Vanilla Pumpkin Seed Clusters

Ingredients
115g (1/2 cup) pumpkin seeds
1 tsp vanilla extract
2 tsp honey
2 tsp coconut sugar
Water (boiled)

Instructions
Preheat oven to 150c.
In a medium bowl, combine the honey, coconut sugar and vanilla. Stir together to create a thick paste then add a small drop of boiled water to thin it out and create a runny syrup.
Pour in the pumpkin seeds and stir them around in the mixture to evenly coat them.
Dollop a generous tsp full of the pumpkin seeds onto a baking sheet, repeat until it's all used up and cook for 15-20 minutes until most of the seeds have browned (but don't let them burn!)
Take out of the oven and leave to cool for a few minutes. Once they've cooled a little (but are still warm) you can press the clusters together to make sure they don't fall apart. They will dry quickly.
Once they're cooled and dried, they're ready to eat! Enjoy on their own or served on top of your cereal.
⏱

188. Almond Joy Sunday

Ingredients
2 cans full fat coconut milk
½ cup honey
1 ½ tablespoons vanilla extract
1 dark baking chocolate bar
¼ cup sliced almonds
½ cup unsweetened coconut flakes

Instructions
In a blender, mix together the coconut milk, honey, and vanilla extract. Line a plastic Tupperware with plastic wrap. Pour the mixture into it and freeze it overnight. The next day, take half of the frozen mixture and add it to a food processor. Mix it on high until it resembles frozen yogurt and put it back into a storage container.
Repeat this process with the other half of the mixture.
Return the blended ice cream to the freeze for 30 minutes before serving.
To assemble, melt the chocolate chips in a saucepan over low heat, to prevent burning the chocolate.
Serve each Almond Joy Sunday with a scoop of the ice cream.
Drizzle the melted chocolate on top, then sprinkle with coconut flakes and sliced almonds. Serve immediately.
⁇

189. Spiced Autumn Apples Baked in Brandy

Ingredients
2 apples of your choice (I used gala, but choose your favourite!)
1 cup brandy
1/4 cup walnuts
1/4 cup raisins
1/4 tablespoon nutmeg
1/4 tablespoon cinnamon
1/4 tablespoon ground cloves

Instructions
Preheat oven to 350 degrees Fahrenheit.
Slice the very top and very bottom off of each apple. (The top allows for more room to stuff with goodies, the bottom allows the apples to soak up all the nice sauce).
Core both apples to the bottom, but not all the way through.
Mix brandy, spices, walnuts, and raisins in a small bowl.
Pour half of the brandy spice mixture into each apple.
Place on baking sheet and bake 20-25 minutes, or until apples are soft. I like to pour any remaining sauce mixture into the bottom of the pan so the apples can soak up the flavours.
Serve and enjoy! My roommate enjoyed his with a side of vanilla coconut milk ice cream.

Notes
Recipe makes 2 servings
Nutrition Facts Per Serving
Calories: 353
Total Fat: 10.0g
Saturated Fat: 0.6g
Carbs: 32.4g
Fiber: 4.0g
Protein: 4.6g
⍰

190. Chocolate Bavarian Cheesecake

Ingredients
For the base:
15 Easy Chocolate Cookies
¼ cup coconut oil (melted)
OR
2 cups nuts
1 cup dried dates (soaked in water)

For the middle:
2+1/2 cups raw cashews (soaked in water for 6 or more hours)
½ cup honey
¼ cup coconut oil
¼ cup cacao powder
½ cup coconut milk
½ cup orange juice

For the top:
1 can coconut cream (chilled in fridge overnight)
Cacao nibs to decorate

Instructions
For the base:
Grind the chocolate cookies in a food processor until fine. Add the melted coconut oil and process until mixture sticks together. Add another tablespoon of coconut oil if you need to.
Press the crumbs into the base of a 21cm springform tin. If you don't have a springform tin, just line your tin with plastic wrap or baking paper so you can remove it easily.
OR
If you can't be bothered making the cookies (or didn't have any in the freezer like I did), just process 2 cups of nuts in a food processor until finely chopped. (Any combination of nuts works well. I've tried just macadamias and it is beautiful and also a combination of cashews, macadamias, hazelnuts, walnuts and brazil nuts)
When your nuts are finely chopped, drain the soaked dates, getting out as much water as you can. Then add them to the food processor and process until it makes a sticky dough.
Next, scoop the date & nut mixture into your pan. Put small plastic freezer bags onto your hands and use your fingers to spread the mixture evenly into the pan. (No sticky fingers!)

For the filling:

Drain the cashews well. Put all of the filling ingredients into a high speed blender or processor and process until smooth. I have a new Froothie blender that is amazing! I compared it to the Vita Mix and it's cheaper and more powerful. You know I love a bargain. Anyway, I'm really happy with it and it makes amazing cheesecake filling!

You will need to use the tamper if you have one and regularly scrape down the sides to make sure all the ingredients are blended together. Keep processing until it is super smooth. Lots of taste testing needed for this step!

Once the mixture is smooth, scrape it all into your pan, on top of the base mixture. Spread it out with a spatula.

Cover with plastic wrap, then put into the freezer for at least 6 hours to set.

When ready to serve, take it from the freezer and defrost for around 30 minutes to soften slightly before cutting. (15 mins for minis.)

While it's defrosting, beat the cream that rises to the top of the coconut cream after it's been refrigerated. Use electric beaters and add some honey to taste if you like.

Spread or pipe the cream over the top of your cheesecake and decorate with cacao nibs.

☐

191. Raw Brownie Bites

Ingredients
1 1/2 cups walnuts
Pinch of salt
1 cup pitted dates
1 tsp vanilla
1/3 cup unsweetened cocoa powder

Instructions
Add walnuts and salt to a blender or food processor. Mix until the walnuts are finely ground.
Add the dates, vanilla, and cocoa powder to the blender. Mix well until everything is combined. With the blender still running, add a couple drops of water at a time to make the mixture stick together.
Using a spatula, transfer the mixture into a bowl. Using your hands, form small round balls, rolling in your palm. Store in an airtight container in the refrigerator for up to a week.

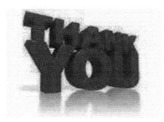

Before you go

I am so delighted that you have chosen this book and it's been a pleasure writing it for you. My mission is to help as many readers as possible to benefit from the content you have just been reading. So many of us are able to take new information and apply it to our lives with really positive and long lasting consequences and it is my wish that you have been able to take value from the information I have presented.

Thank you for staying with me during this book and for reading it through to the end. I really hope that you have enjoyed the contents and that's why I appreciate your feedback so much. If you could take a couple of minutes to review the book, your views will help me to create more material that you find beneficial.

Thanks again for your support and encouragement. I really look forward to reading your review.

Stay Healthy!

To write your review please go to the Amazon Book Page

Made in the USA
Columbia, SC
20 June 2022

61973896R00122